W0234542

▶ **Regulating Preimplantation Genetic Diagnosis in the United States**

DOI: 10.1057/9781137515445.0001

Palgrave Series in Bioethics and Public Policy

Series Editor: **Sheldon Krimsky**, the Lenore Stern Professor of Humanities and Social Sciences and Adjunct Professor of Public Health and Community Medicine at Tufts University, USA.

Professor Krimsky is the author, co-author, and editor of fourteen books including *Genetic Justice: DNA Databanks, Criminal Investigations and Civil Liberties*, awarded a gold medal by the Independent Publishers in 2011. Professor Krimsky served on the National Institutes of Health's Recombinant DNA Advisory Committee and was a consultant to the Presidential Commission for the Study of Ethical Problems in Medicine and Biomedical and Behavioral Research and to the Congressional Office of Technology Assessment. Recently, he served as associate editor, for *Bioethics, 2014*, a reference volume for the field.

Biotechnology continues to impact populations in myriad ways-influencing contemporary issues in food supply, genetic therapy, health care, biosecurity, terrorism, criminal justice, food supply, and environmental engineering among many other aspects of daily life. The *Palgrave Series in Bioethics and Public Policy* seeks to promote interdisciplinary research that analyzes and assesses the social, environmental, and moral ramifications of where this technology is taking us. With a wide range of topics within bioethics open to the series, this series will provide a home for cutting-edge research that bridges the divide between the natural and social sciences. This series will also attract a dynamic and varied assortment of scholars to provide comprehensive evaluations of where biotechnology is taking our society-and most importantly, if these directions are being forged appropriately and ethically.

Titles include:

Michelle Bayefsky and Bruce Jennings
REGULATING PREIMPLANTATION GENETIC DIAGNOSIS IN THE UNITED STATES
The Limits of Unlimited Selection

DOI: 10.1057/9781137515445.0001

palgrave▸pivot

Regulating Preimplantation Genetic Diagnosis in the United States: The Limits of Unlimited Selection

Michelle Bayefsky

and

Bruce Jennings

palgrave
macmillan

DOI: 10.1057/9781137515445.0001

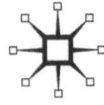

REGULATING PREIMPLANTATION GENETIC DIAGNOSIS IN THE UNITED STATES

Copyright © Michelle Bayefsky and Bruce Jennings, 2015.

All rights reserved.

First published in 2015 by
PALGRAVE MACMILLAN®
in the United States—a division of St. Martin's Press LLC,
175 Fifth Avenue, New York, NY 10010.

Where this book is distributed in the UK, Europe and the rest of the world, this is by Palgrave Macmillan, a division of Macmillan Publishers Limited, registered in England, company number 785998, of Houndmills, Basingstoke, Hampshire RG21 6XS.

Palgrave Macmillan is the global academic imprint of the above companies and has companies and representatives throughout the world.

Palgrave® and Macmillan® are registered trademarks in the United States, the United Kingdom, Europe and other countries.

ISBN: 978–1–137–51545–2 EPUB
ISBN: 978–1–137–51544–5 PDF
ISBN: 978–1–137–51543–8 Hardback

Library of Congress Cataloging-in-Publication Data is available from the Library of Congress.

A catalogue record of the book is available from the British Library.

First edition: 2015

www.palgrave.com/pivot

DOI: 10.1057/9781137515445

Contents

Acknowledgments   vii

1   Introduction   1
Preimplantation genetic diagnosis:
    the technique and its uses   3
PGD practice in the United States   6
Ethical controversies: an overview   7
The regulation of PGD   11
Health care financing and coverage of PGD   12

2   The Ethics of PGD and Its Relevance to
    Regulation   18
The ethical critique of PGD: mastery
    and acceptance   20
Parental duties and the genetic shaping of
    children   24
The ethical case for PGD: procreative
    beneficence   31

3   Drawing Ethical Lines   39
Defining disease   40
Selecting against deafness   44
Selecting for deafness   48
Adult onset diseases   50
Savior siblings: creating one life for the
    sake of another   52
Elective sex selection   54

4   Regulating PGD in Practice   59
Reproductive autonomy and Its limits   60

Eugenics and its implications for PGD   65
Options for regulation   68
Summary: the pros and cons of government
    regulation vs. professional self-regulation   77
Regulatory flexibility in scientific and moral
    gray areas: the example of the HFEA   79
Who should decide?   81
The bottom line   82

5 Paying for PGD   89
   Conclusion   96

Bibliography   100

Index   110

Acknowledgments

We wish to thank Professor Stephen Latham (Director, Yale Interdisciplinary Center for Bioethics) for his advice and support, and for carefully reading and commenting on a draft of this book. We are also grateful to those who agreed to be interviewed, and whose insights and opinions we have included. Specifically (in chronological order), we thank Dr Mark Hughes, Founder and Director of Genesis Genetics; Dr Paula Amato, Chair of the Ethics Committee of the American Society for Reproductive Medicine; Dr Santiago Munné, Founder and Director of Reprogenetics; Ms Barbara Collura, President and CEO of RESOLVE; Professor Anita Silvers, Chair of Philosophy at San Francisco State University; Professor Laura Mauldin, Assistant Professor in the Women's, Gender and Sexuality Studies, Department of the University of Connecticut; Professor Leslie Francis, Distinguished Professor of Philosophy, Associate Dean for Faculty Research and Development at the University of Utah College of Law; and Ms Alison Lashwood, Clinical Lead in PGD at the Centre for Preimplantation Genetic Diagnosis at Guy's and St Thomas' Hospital in London, England. In addition, we would like to express our appreciation to those who shared with us their wisdom and understanding of the field over the course of our research. In particular, we would like to thank Dr Thomas Murray, President Emeritus and Senior Research Scholar of The Hastings Center for Bioethics; Professor Arthur Caplan, Director of NYU Langone Division of Medical Ethics; Dr Dan Goldschlag, OB/GYN and specialist in reproductive endocrinology and infertility at the Weill Cornell Center for Reproductive Medicine; Dr Pasquale Patrizio, OB/GYN and specialist in reproductive endocrinology and infertility at the Yale Fertility Center; Ms Lee Rubin-Collins, former board member and volunteer at RESOLVE; Ms Kristin MacCutcheon, PGD nurse coordinator at the Boston IVF Clinic; and Ms Marymichele Delaney, Associate Director of Benefits at Wellesley.

DOI: 10.1057/9781137515445.0002

1
Introduction

Abstract: *In this chapter, we lay out the potential and actual uses of preimplantation genetic diagnosis (PGD). We include an explanation of the medical process and current limitations of reproductive medicine and genetic sequencing technology, as well as a presentation of existing empirical data on the use of PGD in the United States. We then briefly summarize the ethical dilemmas surrounding various uses of PGD, including nonmedical sex selection, selection against adult onset diseases, selection for a tissue match for a sick sibling, and selection for a disability such as deafness. The chapter also includes a description of the current regulatory landscape for PGD in the United States as compared to two Western European countries (the UK and France), and ends with a discussion of the relationships between health care financing in the United States, insurance coverage of PGD, and the current dearth of regulation.*

Bayefsky, Michelle and Bruce Jennings. *Regulating Preimplantation Genetic Diagnosis in the United States: The Limits of Unlimited Selection.* New York: Palgrave Macmillan, 2015. DOI: 10.1057/9781137515445.0003.

As science and medicine rapidly advance, philosophers, social scientists, and policymakers struggle to apply ethical and policy frameworks to the use of new technologies. Ordinary citizens also struggle with the moral, religious, and personal implications of biotechnology. Sometimes, as with human reproductive cloning, there is a strong public response, numerous state bans, and a general consensus that a particular procedure is deeply problematic from an ethical and social point of view. Other times, as with stem cell research, public opinion is divided on the question of whether the application is acceptable, and the government intervenes to draw moral lines in the sand and restrict public funding for research. In yet other situations, the public is undereducated, federal and state governments are silent (or paralyzed), and medical technology continues to advance relatively unfettered by moral and regulatory restraints.

This latter pattern has been the case in the United States with the technology that is the subject of this book: preimplantation genetic diagnosis (PGD). PGD is a procedure performed on embryos following *in vitro* fertilization (IVF) or on polar bodies (to preclude an X linked disorder) in order to obtain genetic information prior to uterine implantation. Couples wishing to benefit from PGD may decide to go through the process of IVF even though they are not infertile. Normally, several embryos are created for PGD and some are selected for transfer into the uterus, while others are discarded, including those in which no genetic abnormality was found.[1] Although the ethical dilemmas and implications surrounding the use of PGD are significant and have been the subject of scholarly exploration, the technology continues to be unregulated by either federal or state law.

PGD was first successfully used in 1989 as an alternative to prenatal genetic testing, which can pose an anguishing decision concerning abortion. Initially, it was designed to identify a small number of serious genetic disorders that would cause chronic illness and/or foreshorten life (such as cystic fibrosis, fragile X, beta thalassemia, Tay-Sachs, and sickle cell anemia). But as genetic science and technology have advanced, PGD has come to be used for a broader range of conditions and purposes. PGD thus raises a number of provocative bioethical issues that are both philosophical and ethical, including the definition of disease, the specter of eugenics, the rights of parents to decide the genetic makeup of their children and governments to restrict the procreative freedom of its citizens. Even beyond these powerful questions, PGD differs from

DOI: 10.1057/9781137515445.0003

other controversial innovations in medical technology in its ability to impact the future of our species. By testing embryos' genes and choosing to implant some embryos rather than others, doctors and scientists make permanent changes in the genetic makeup of future generations. Given the far-reaching consequences of this technology, it is imperative that we carefully examine the ethical implications of its various potential applications before deciding whether and how to restrict its use.

This book will explore the numerous ethical issues surrounding the use of PGD. Rather than attempting to resolve these moral issues or end debate, however, we aim to lay out the competing values and moral views at stake. Above all, we focus on the question of the governance of genetic technology in the case of PGD: should PGD be regulated in the United States, and if so, how could this be done in the context of current medical, political, and economic realities? We do not take this current context to be immutable, however, as it reflects the views and interests of the relevant stakeholders and the general populace, and these factors are contingent and dynamic. Our analysis will draw upon interviews with fertility specialists, patient advocates, philosophers, and representatives of physicians' associations, along with survey data on the public's views on PGD. Our goal is to provide an account of the pertinent ethical questions, the regulatory options in the current practice of PGD, and the barriers to developing regulations for PGD in the United States.

Preimplantation genetic diagnosis: the technique and its uses

Preimplantation genetic diagnosis is the technique used during *in vitro* fertilization (IVF) to check an embryo's genes for heritable conditions. Prospective parents[2] who know that they are carriers of a particular heritable disease, such as cystic fibrosis, can choose to undergo fertility treatment in order to guarantee that the disease will not be passed on to their child. Alternatively, they may conceive a child naturally, screen the fetus genetically via chorionic villus sampling at week 10 or amniocentesis at week 16, and decide whether to terminate the pregnancy if the fetus tests positive for the disease. The decision to have an abortion can be very difficult, and using PGD to select for a healthy embryo allows couples at risk for having a child with a genetic disease to avoid recourse to abortion.

DOI: 10.1057/9781137515445.0003

In order to utilize PGD, a couple must go through an IVF cycle, which involves several steps. After consultation with a fertility specialist, the woman self-administers daily hormone injections in order to stimulate her ovaries to produce multiple eggs, rather than a single egg per ovulatory cycle. She comes in for check-ups every two—three days and a doctor or nurse performs transvaginal ultrasounds in order to monitor the growth of the eggs and time the egg retrieval. When the eggs are ready to be retrieved, the woman takes additional hormones to trigger ovulation. Then, under general anesthesia or a combination of local anesthesia and sedation, her doctor collects the eggs from follicles which have reached the size that typically indicates maturity (18–22 mm in diameter). The egg retrieval involves using transvaginal ultrasound to guide a needle through the wall of the vagina into the ovary, where the fluid within each follicle is aspirated.[3]

Next, an embryologist examines the content of the aspirated fluid and fertilizes the eggs that have indeed reached maturity with sperm collected from the patient's partner or a donor. To perform PGD, the resulting embryos are incubated for two—three days and then one or two cells are taken for DNA testing. One or more embryos that are deemed healthy after genetic testing are subsequently transferred into the uterus.[4] If the any of the embryos successfully implants in the uterus, the woman becomes pregnant.

While PGD was originally intended for couples seeking to avoid passing on a genetic disease, the capacity to screen embryos prior to implantation lends itself to uses apart from having a healthy child. For example, couples in which one or both partners are deaf or of very short stature (dwarfism) have asked fertility specialists in the United States to use PGD to select *for* a child with deafness or dwarfism.[5] Furthermore, parents of sick children in need of a stem cell transplant but unable to find a suitable donor have done PGD in order to give birth to a child who can serve as a tissue match for his or her sibling (a "savior sibling"). This application is known as Human Leukocyte Antigen (HLA) typing, after the antigen that must match the sick sibling's antigens in order for a stem cell donation from the younger child's (sometimes referred to as the "savior sibling") umbilical cord blood to be accepted.[6]

In the United States, the most common uses of PGD are for the purpose of selecting an embryo without a specific genetic disease for implantation. However, PGD is also relatively commonly used for the purpose of elective sex selection.[7] Couples seeking to have a child of a

DOI: 10.1057/9781137515445.0003

preferred sex can utilize IVF techniques even when they are not infertile, and they can have PGD performed so that only the embryos of the preferred sex will be transferred into the woman's uterus. Finally, as our ability to sequence DNA rapidly and test for specific genes advances, it will be possible to use PGD to select for and against an even wider range of conditions or even certain traits.

Recent developments in genetic sequencing technology render the possibility of greatly expanding the conditions for which PGD is used extremely probable, if not inevitable. In January 2014, Illumina, Inc., the world's leading seller of gene sequencing technology, released a next-generation sequencing tool called the NextSeq 500 System, which can sequence a whole human genome in one day. Illumina's portfolio of sequencers also includes the HiSeq X sequencer, which is the world's first system to sequence whole genomes for under $1,000.[8] Fertility centers and laboratories are already using next-generation whole-genome sequencing as a more cost effective and reliable way to perform preimplantation chromosomal screening (PGS) or single-gene PGD.[9]

In addition to having the scientific capacity to use advanced genetic sequencing technology for PGD, doctors and scientists now have the FDA's implicit approval. In December 2013, the FDA approved Illumina's next-generation MiSeqDx system, which was designed specifically for clinical laboratories. In a perspective piece in the *New England Journal of Medicine*, FDA Commissioner Margaret Hamburg and NIH Director Francis Collins highlighted the significance of this development, writing that FDA approval will allow "any lab to test any sequence for any purpose."[10] PGD will surely be one of the many genetic techniques that are revolutionized by rapid whole-genome sequencing.

Next-generation sequencing will be attractive to fertility specialists and patients in need of PGD due to its ever-decreasing costs, accuracy, and speed. Currently, patients who use PGD must wait a whole month to transfer embryos to the uterus because after the embryos resulting from IVF are biopsied, they must be cryopreserved so that they do not develop beyond the optimal point for implantation while the genetic tests are being run.[11] These tests generally take about one week, so if the embryos are biopsied on day 2 or 3 after fertilization and need to be transferred by day 5 or 6, they must be frozen before the results of the genetic tests are returned.[12] By the time the results are in, the woman's uterine lining is no longer receptive to implantation and so the couple must wait for her next menstrual cycle in order to transfer the healthy embryos. If PGD can

DOI: 10.1057/9781137515445.0003

be performed within 24 hours, cryopreservation of the embryos would not be necessary, and the whole process could be completed within one month. This may be attractive to couples for many reasons, including avoiding the potential risks of cryopreservation.

Although PGD will likely be performed using advanced genetic screening technology, including whole-genome sequencing, relatively soon, limitations in genomics, reproductive medicine, and perhaps even biology itself will prevent new sequencing capacities from being used to select for a wide range of diseases and traits in the near future. In genomics, scientists have yet to uncover the genes that code for many conditions, or all of the different genes that contribute to particular traits. In reproductive medicine, an average IVF cycle will produce approximately six embryos of high enough quality (at the blastocyst stage) to transfer to the uterus. This is not enough for a couple trying to select for or against several traits, let alone traits coded by hundreds of genes (e.g. intelligence).[13] The limitation in reproductive medicine lies in specialists' inability to stimulate the ovaries to produce a large number of eggs for retrieval without causing hyperstimulation of the ovaries, which is dangerous and painful for the patient. It would take scores or even hundreds of eggs to produce enough embryos for parents to have a significant selective capacity. Scientists are working to develop a technique for using excised ovarian tissue to develop mature eggs *in vitro*, which could allow for the production of many eggs at one time while circumventing the problem of hyperstimulation. However, this research is in its early stages,[14] and the selective capacity of patients and doctors currently remains limited. Furthermore, it is unclear to what extent genetic manipulation can be used to select certain traits anyhow, since environmental factors play an important role in the development of phenotypes and behaviors.

PGD practice in the United States

Data on the use of PGD in the United States are limited. The Society for Assisted Reproductive Technology (SART), an organization of reproductive medical professionals affiliated with the American Society of Reproductive Medicine, analyzes annual data collected by the CDC from approximately 95% of fertility clinics nationwide and reports IVF outcomes by measures such as "percentage of cycles resulting in

DOI: 10.1057/9781137515445.0003

pregnancy" and "percentage of cycles resulting in live births."[15] The data collected include the number of IVF cycles that incorporate PGD, but not why PGD was performed. In the most recent data to be released, from 2012, 5% of IVF cycles nationwide (of a total of 165,172 cycles) were "PGD cycles."[16] For 2007 and 2008, however, SART researchers collected somewhat more detailed data on the use of PGD. In 2008, they found that 4.2% of all IVF cycles were PGD cycles, and of that 4.2%, 19.8% were for the diagnosis of single-gene disorders such as cystic fibrosis and Tay-Sachs, 52.3% were for aneuploidy screening (PGS), and 20.3% were for elective sex selection.[17]

The other major source of data on the use of PGD in the United States is a study published by Susannah Baruch, J.D., David Kaufman, Ph.D. and Kathy Hudson, Ph.D. from Johns Hopkins University's Genetics and Public Policy Center (GPPC) in 2006. The GPPC researchers submitted an 87-question survey on PGD practices to 415 US fertility clinics. Of the 415, 190 clinics responded and 186 of them performed PGD. They found that of the PGD cycles performed in 2005, 66% were for aneuploidy screening, 12% were for the diagnosis of single-gene disorders, 1% were for HLA matching, and 9% were for nonmedical sex selection. Additionally, 3% of IVF-PGD clinics reported performing PGD to select *for* a disability such as deafness.[18]

The GPPC numbers differ from those collected by SART; specifically, the percentages of PGD cycles performed for elective sex selection and the diagnosis of single-gene disorders are higher in the SART study. It is unclear whether these differences arise from changing practices between 2005 and 2008 or differences in the way the researchers collected their data. Furthermore, these data may have limited applicability since both datasets are over five years old and PGD practices might have shifted in recent years as genetic technology has advanced and more people have learned about the procedure's availability. Nevertheless, both datasets indicate that PGD has been used in the United States for a variety of medical and nonmedical purposes.

Ethical controversies: an overview

Given the technique's current and potential capacity to select for children with and without particular characteristics, PGD has been a controversial medical tool.[19] The different applications of PGD are surrounded by

DOI: 10.1057/9781137515445.0003

varying levels of controversy and can be characterized in different ways. Susannah Baruch divides the applications of PGD into four basic categories. According to her analysis, PGD can either be used to select against fatal or severe diseases, or to suit parental preferences by performing (1) HLA matching to save an older child, (2) selection against adult-onset disease, (3) nonmedical sex selection, or (4) selection *for* a disability.[20] In a subsequent study, she reports that PGD to select against severe diseases such as Tay-Sachs or cystic fibrosis is relatively uncontroversial in the United States, though there is no consensus on what constitutes a serious or severe disease.[21] Each of these four uses of PGD raises ethical issues.[22]

HLA matching is meant to supply umbilical cord blood from a new child to a sick sibling for use in stem cell transplantation. Sometimes PGD is already necessary for the second child to ensure that he or she does not share the hereditary illness of his or her sibling, but other times PGD is done solely to find an HLA match, even when there is no risk of hereditary illness to the second child. HLA matching is controversial because creating one child for the sake of another can be interpreted as valuing the second child only instrumentally and treating that child primarily as a means to save the life or promote the health of the older child. Is this a failure to respect the human dignity of the younger child? Does it violate a core obligation of parents, who should have equal moral regard for each of their children? Does it constitute a misuse of ART and PGD? Furthermore, this application raises ethical questions relating to the need to prevent harm and promote the best interests of a child. Thus far, studies have indicated that PGD is not associated with increased risks of low birth weight, premature birth, serious abnormalities, and perinatal death compared with other IVF-newborns.[23] However, there are no reliable long-term data on the effects of PGD.[24] Thus for both reasons of human rights and dignity and for reasons of promoting the well-being and best interests of all children, we must consider the ethical implications of subjecting a later child to unforeseen long-term consequences for the sake of an existing sibling.

PGD can also be performed for a wide range of adult-onset diseases, or diseases that only manifest themselves in adulthood. These include breast cancer, Huntington's disease, and perhaps in the future, certain genetically associated forms of Alzheimer's disease.[25] The example of Huntington's, an autosomal dominant genetic disorder, is perhaps most straightforward due to its high degree of expressivity and penetrance. Huntington's is such a debilitating disease that many persons who have

DOI: 10.1057/9781137515445.0003

this genetic allele refrain from procreation, or at least are very troubled by the decision to risk having an affected child. It is clear that guaranteeing through PGD that a child will not be at risk for Huntington's would be extremely beneficial to the child, both in youth and adulthood. In this instance, the use of PGD is not ethically controversial. Other genetic risk factors, however, such as breast cancer, are more uncertain, and if disease does manifest later in life it may be medically treatable or have a less dramatic effect on the length and quality of a person's life. An increased genetic risk for breast cancer, for example, can be treated by preventive measures and can be monitored carefully by the patient and her doctor. Thus, while avoiding the risk of breast cancer would offer significant relief to parents and children undergoing PGD, the urgency is somewhat less than in the case of Huntington's, and so the justification for PGD requires more explicit reasoning and argument. Even if reliable genetic markers could be discovered for a wide range of common chronic illnesses and late onset conditions, such as heart disease, type II diabetes, and osteoarthritis, would it be feasible and desirable to use PGD to prevent them? Those born with genetic factors associated with increased risk for late onset conditions still live a long, full life, one comparable to those who develop those illnesses without genetic abnormalities. Using genetic factors to decide whether or not to begin a human life is the essence of PGD. Judgments about the quality of life (as well as questions about the predictive power of genetics) are unavoidable. Using PGD to select against some adult-onset diseases leans in the direction of utilizing a powerful medical tool to create children that have particular advantages, or suit parental preferences, rather than out of absolute necessity.

Nonmedical sex selection, or selection of a child of a particular sex for reasons unrelated to the transmission of a sex-linked disease, is likewise ethically problematic because of its use of PGD to suit parental preferences. Is it morally acceptable for parents to view their children as genetic products to be chosen, in some sense? Does this kind of mentality detract from the unconditional love that we value in parent–child relationships? Does choosing a child's genes differ from raising a child in accordance with parental values and preferences? If so, how?

Some also object to elective sex selection on the grounds that it may create a gender disparity, like the gap created in China through selective abortion under the one-child policy.[26] Thus sex selection might not only reinforce gender bias at a familial level, but also on a societal level.[27]

DOI: 10.1057/9781137515445.0003

Evidence on PGD for sex selection in the United States suggests that there is no preference for one specific gender in couples of Western origin, but certain minority populations such as those of Chinese, Indian, and Middle-Eastern origin exhibit a preference for males.[28] Given the relatively small percentage of people in the United States from China, India, or the Middle East and the small scale on which PGD is performed, elective sex selection using PGD is unlikely to cause a demographic shift.[29] Nevertheless, for families of non-Western origin with particular gender preferences, using PGD for sex selection reinforces those biases, potentially to the detriment of female members of those populations in the United States.

The final category, PGD to select *for* a particular disability, or more precisely, for particular genetic traits, is also morally questionable because of its use of reproductive medical technology to create a child suited to parental preferences. It is also questionable due to the complexity of determining whether doing so would be in the "best interests" of the child. Here the question of what constitutes a "disability" is important. The practice is relatively uncommon (only 3% of fertility clinics reported providing this service in the GPPC study), but nevertheless worthy of attention given its permissibility in the United States.[30] Parents with deafness or dwarfism are motivated by legitimate concerns about having a child that will fit in with their communities and lifestyles. However, by choosing to have a child with a disability, the parents are putting that child at a disadvantage by some social metrics, and an argument can be made that the parents are limiting the future child's autonomy. This argument is contentious, however, since it entails value judgments about life with a disability as compared to life without a disability, as well as how to define "disability" to begin with. Philosophical work in this area has also centered on the "non-identity" problem, or the difficulty that the alternative for the child born with a disability after undergoing PGD is not to have been born at all.

Beyond concerns about the meaning of parenthood, the autonomy of the future child, and the potential for reinforcing biases are questions about the limits of human power and whether we ought to tinker with nature in this manner. Some feel intuitively uncomfortable with the level of control we are exerting over human life and nature by selecting for some genes over others. While this intuition is difficult to translate into a consistent regulatory framework, it should not be disregarded in a discussion of the ethics of regulating PGD.

DOI: 10.1057/9781137515445.0003

The regulation of PGD

In the United States, there are few state or federal laws on assisted reproductive technology (ART) and there are no laws whatsoever on the various uses of PGD.[31] Bioethicist Arthur Caplan has gone as far as to call reproductive medicine the "Wild West" of medicine today.[32] Professional self-regulation by physicians' associations including the American Society for Reproductive Medicine (ASRM), the American College of Medical Genetics (ACMG), and the American Congress of Obstetricians and Gynecologists (ACOG) is the primary means by which the uses of PGD are regulated, and these associations offer minimal and often open-ended guidance on PGD. Furthermore, professional self-regulation is not legally binding, though physicians' societies' guidelines are cited by insurance companies weighing what procedures to cover and courts deciding whether a doctor has breached the standard of care in his or her medical field.

The regulatory landscape of ART and PGD in the United States is very different from other Western countries. For example, in the United Kingdom, the National Health Service (NHS) and a statutory body called the "Human Fertilisation and Embryology Authority" (HFEA) carefully regulate what assisted-reproductive technologies may be legally offered and are covered by the single-payer system. The HFEA receives its authority from two pieces of national legislation—the Human Fertilisation and Embryology Acts of 1990 and 2008. These bills explicitly allow for the use of ART for heterosexual couples, homosexual couples, and single women. Paid surrogacy is prohibited, gamete donation may not be anonymous, and PGD can only be used for medical purposes. The "medical purposes" of PGD include HLA antigen-matching to select for a child who will serve as a donor for a sick sibling (although the medical purpose is not directly related to the health of the resulting child). PGD for sex selection is only permitted when a couple is attempting to select against a sex-linked disorder; elective sex selection is illegal.[33] The HFEA has a detailed list of disorders for which PGD is permitted,[34] which is updated as patients apply for new conditions to be added to the list.

Another example of careful regulation of ART is in France, where ART is only allowed for heterosexual couples in which the woman is under 43 years of age, since homosexual couples and single and older women are not considered *medically* infertile. The emphasis on using medical technology to solve medical problems is extended to PGD, where like the

UK, the procedure may only be used to select against specific diseases or to select for an HLA antigen match.[35] A French government agency created by France's 2004 Bioethics Law, the Agence de la Biomédecine, is charged with overseeing several areas in human biology and medicine, including assisted-reproductive medicine and PGD. The Agence has published ethics opinions and reports on PGD practices and has the power to extend the uses of PGD laid out in the 1994, 2004, and 2011 French bioethics laws.

Without this kind of governmental regulation, access to ART in the United States is not restricted for homosexual couples, single people, or older patients. At the same time, there are no legal limitations on the different uses of PGD. As a result, as mentioned earlier, current uses of PGD in the United States include nonmedical sex selection and selection for certain disabilities such as dwarfism and deafness. Chapter 4 will explore justifications for regulating the various uses of PGD. How should we address the question of whether PGD regulations are necessary at present? If they are, who should be responsible for regulating PGD? Is the current state of professional self-regulation sufficient? How can we regulate a medical technology when such a plurality of opinions exists on what uses are ethical? Chapters 4 and 5 will incorporate available data on public opinion about PGD, several proposals on how PGD might be regulated, and interviews with stakeholders including patient advocates, fertility specialists, bioethicists, and representatives of the relevant physicians' associations.

Health care financing and coverage of PGD

In a single-payer insurance system, the regulation of medical services can be leveraged through government financing policies. This is not the case in the domain of reproductive medicine in the United States today. Other mechanisms of reproductive technology governance must be used, such as legislation, administrative regulation, licensure, and civil court actions.

Hence, the lack of regulation of ART in the United States can be explained in part by the limitations placed on direct government involvement in most forms of health care financing in the United States. Direct government funding for health care takes place through Medicare (for the elderly and severely disabled), Medicaid (for low-income recipients and some long-term care services), and the Department of Veterans

DOI: 10.1057/9781137515445.0003

Affairs system. However, advanced ART procedures such as IVF are not covered through these schemes, so the government has not been required to develop guidelines for the appropriate coverage of IVF or PGD.

Many Americans receive health care benefits through employer-sponsored insurance, and beginning in 2014 under the Affordable Care Act, virtually all individuals not otherwise insured must purchase individual coverage from private companies through competitive market exchanges set up by state and the Federal government for this purpose. Thus one way or another, a large majority of Americans receive health care funding through private insurance companies. In the absence of a mandate requiring coverage for a particular procedure (there is no such mandate for PGD), there is wide variation in the benefits offered by insurance plans and in the procedures and services that are covered and to what extent. Moreover, private insurers are concerned with the cost of services but do not have authority to regulate the quality and delivery of services such as PGD or ART. Therefore, the reliance on private insurance companies in the United States means that there is no automatic need for a government agency to determine what applications of PGD to permit in order to decide what uses to fund.

By contrast, the United Kingdom has the publicly funded National Health Service (NHS). The NHS directly employs most doctors, and other doctors have contracts with their local Clinical Commissioning Groups (CCGs). CCGs are local trusts overseen by the NHS responsible for deciding exactly what services are needed and ensuring that they are provided.[36] The trusts will only cover the uses of PGD approved by the HFEA, so it is necessary for the HFEA to have a system for determining which conditions to approve. Similarly, France has a system of universal health care in which the government-funded National Health Insurance (NHI) pays for 73% of all medical spending and the rest is covered by supplemental private insurers and patient co-payments.[37] Since the NHI insurance will cover PGD, it must have clear guidelines for what applications of PGD to cover.

Theoretically, Medicaid, which is federally funded, would require a list of approved uses of PGD. (Medicare is also federally funded but is primarily applicable for post-menopausal women.) However, Medicaid does not list infertility services as one of its essential health benefits[38] and thus state Medicaid plans are not required to offer fertility services. For example, Connecticut's Medicaid services include the diagnosis of infertility but no infertility treatment.[39] Thus, there has been no need for a federal or state-approved list of conditions for which PGD should be used.

DOI: 10.1057/9781137515445.0003

Despite the lack of government involvement in payment for PGD, private health insurance companies do offer plans that include coverage of PGD. However, they often do not cover IVF, since only 15 states require health insurance companies to cover any kind of fertility treatment. Three of these states specifically exclude coverage of IVF, and other states have difficult standards for meeting the state's definition of "infertile" (e.g. Hawaii, which requires that a couple try and fail to get pregnant for five years).[40] Even in states which require that insurance companies cover at least one cycle of IVF, a couple in need of PGD would not meet the criteria for infertility if the members are fully capable of getting pregnant but have a genetic condition they hope to avoid passing on. Couples in need of PGD fall through the insurance cracks because they are not technically infertile, but they still need to use fertility services in order to have healthy children. Thus their options include feigning infertility by claiming to have tried to have a child for the requisite period of time[41] or paying around $12,000 per cycle to cover the costs of IVF out of pocket, and then asking their insurance company to cover the $3,550 cost of PGD.[42]

In Chapter 5, we will discuss insurance coverage for PGD in greater depth, as well as several pros and cons of providing coverage for IVF and PGD from an insurance company's point of view. It is important to keep in mind, however, that while the various uses of PGD may be limited for some by what applications are covered by insurance, without government regulation, those who can afford it will continue to be able to pay out of pocket for uses of PGD that are not approved by insurance companies.

As we now embark on a more detailed discussion of the ethics, regulation, and financing of PGD, we should keep in mind that all these dimensions must be considered simultaneously in order to gain a complete picture of the governance of PGD and of the benefits and drawbacks of regulations concerning its access and use. Ethics infuses political and economic considerations on the various uses of PGD, and political and economic considerations influence the expression and prioritization of ethical viewpoints.

Notes

1   One aspect of the ethical issues raised by PGD concerns proper respect for and handling of human embryos *in vitro*. The fact that some embryos that

do not have genetic abnormalities are discarded, if they are not frozen or donated, is a complicated issue, but it is not one that we shall focus on in this study. For a discussion, see Batzer and Ravitsky, 2009.

2   In this description, we refer to "prospective parents" and "the couple" since reproductive partners most often are involved in the use of PGD and make joint decisions regarding it. We recognize, of course, that this procedure, like other forms of assisted reproductive technology (ART), may be used by an individual woman to achieve pregnancy and to manage its course. We also recognize that the decision to terminate a pregnancy in the light of PGD or prenatal genetic testing is the legal prerogative of the pregnant woman.

3   "Egg Retrieval and Embryo Transfer." *Preparing for Egg Retrieval.* Yale Fertility Center, n.d. Web. January 26, 2014 <http://medicine.yale.edu/obgyn/yfc/ourservices/invitro/egg-retrieval.aspx>.

4   "How does PGD Work?" *PGD – Pre-Implantation Genetic Diagnosis (PGD) – Genetic Testing.* Human Fertilisation and Embryology Authority, n.d. Web. November 28, 2013 <http://www.hfea.gov.uk/preimplantation-genetic-diagnosis.html>.

5   Baruch, S. "Preimplantation Genetic Diagnosis and Parental Preferences: Beyond Deadly Disease." *Houston Journal of Health Law & Policy* 8 (2009): 245–270.

6   Ibid.

7   Baruch, S., D. Kaufman, and K. Hudson. "Genetic Testing of Embryos: Practices and Perspectives of US in Vitro Fertilization Clinics." *Fertility and Sterility* 89.5 (2008): 1053–1058.

8   "Illumina Launches the NextSeq(TM) 500 Sequencing System." *Wall Street Journal* [New York City] January 14, 2014.

9   Pers. comm. Dr Mark Hughes, founder and Director of Genesis Genetics, January 15, 2014.

10   Collins, Francis and Margaret Hamburg. "First FDA Authorization for Next-Generation Sequencer." *New England Journal of Medicine* 369.25 (2013).

11   Recent developments in cryopreservation technology have rendered the risk to embryos from freezing and thawing negligible. Still, if the embryos' genes could be sequenced right away, they would avoid the additional procedure of cryopreservation.

12   Braude, Peter, Susan Pickering, Frances Flinter, and Caroline Mackie Ogilvie. "Preimplantation Genetic Diagnosis." *Nature Reviews Genetics* 3.12 (2002): 941–955.

13   Pers. comm. Dr Sanitago Munné, Founder and Director of Reproenetics, January 21, 2014.

14   Huang, Jack, Togas Tulandi, Hananel Holzer, Seang Lin Tan, and Ri-Cheng Chian. "Combining Ovarian Tissue Cryobanking with Retrieval of Immature Oocytes Followed by *in vitro* Maturation and Vitrification: An Additional Strategy of Fertility Preservation." *Fertility and Sterility* 89.3 (2008): 567–572.

DOI: 10.1057/9781137515445.0003

15   Ginsburg, Elizabeth S., Valerie L. Baker, Catherine Racowsky, Ethan
      Wantman, James Goldfarb, and Judy E. Stern. "Use of Preimplantation
      Genetic Diagnosis and Preimplantation Genetic Screening in the United
      States: A Society for Assisted Reproductive Technology Writing Group
      Paper." *Fertility and Sterility* 96.4 (2011): 865–868.

16   "Clinic Summary Report." *SART CORS*. Society for Assisted Reproductive
      Technology, 2012. Web. 11 April, 2014. <https://www.sartcorsonline.com/
      rptCSR_PublicMultYear.aspx?ClinicPKID=0>.

17   Ginsburg *et al.* (2011).

18   Baruch *et al.* (2008) "Genetic Testing of Embryos: Practices and Perspectives
      of US in Vitro Fertilization Clinics."

19   Hudson, K. "Preimplantation Genetic Diagnosis: Public Policy and Public
      Attitudes." *Fertility and Sterility* 85.6 (2006): 1638–1645.

20   Baruch. (2009) "Preimplantation Genetic Diagnosis and Parental
      Preferences: Beyond Deadly Disease."

21   Baruch, Susannah. "PGD: Genetic Testing of Embryos in the United
      States." *JRC European Commission*. Johns Hopkins University, February 15,
      2009. Web. January 26, 2014. <http://ec.europa.eu/dgs/jrc/downloads/
      jrc_aaas_2009_03_baruch_pgd.pdf>.

22   The question of defining disease will be addressed in Chapter 3. Baruch's
      classifications focus on currently available use of PGD, but in later discussion
      we must also consider the use of PGD for enhancement purposes.

23   Gallagher, James. "Preimplantation Genetic Diagnosis for IVF 'is Safe'" *BBC
      News*. BBC, March 7, 2012. Web January 26, 2014. <http://www.bbc.co.uk/
      news/health-18676894>.

24   IVF itself has been associated with a slightly increased risk of birth defects.
      According to the ASRM, the risk of birth defects in children conceived
      naturally is 2–3% whereas the risk of birth defects in children conceived by
      IVF is estimated to be 2.6–3.9% ("Risks of *In Vitro* Fertilization (IVF)." *Patient
      Fact Sheet*. American Society for Reproductive Medicine, Web. April 1, 2014.
      <http://www.asrm.org/Risks_of_In_Vitro_Fertilization_factsheet/>).

25   Baruch, S. (2008) "Preimplantation Genetic Diagnosis and Parental
      Preferences: Beyond Deadly Disease." A single gene related to late onset
      Alzheimer's has not been identified, so it is not yet possible to use PGD for
      this purpose. The genetics of a variant of Alzheimer's that has an earlier onset
      is better understood. For an interesting review of ethical issues, see Post,
      Stephen G. and Whitehouse, Peter J., eds *Genetic Testing for Alzheimer Disease:
      Ethical and Clinical Issues*. Baltimore: The Johns Hopkins University Press,
      1998.

26   LaFraniere, Sharon. "Chinese Bias for Baby Boys Creates a Gap of 32
      Million." *New York Times* April 10, 2009.

DOI: 10.1057/9781137515445.0003

27   Ethics Committee of the American Society for Reproductive Medicine. "Preconception Gender Selection for Nonmedical Reasons." *Fertility and Sterility* 75.5 (2001): 861–864.

28   Colls, P., L. Silver, G. Olivera, J. Weier, T. Escudero, N. Goodall, G. Tomkin, and S. Munné. "Preimplantation Genetic Diagnosis for Gender Selection in the USA." *Reproductive BioMedicine Online* 19 (2009): 16–22.

29   Ibid.

30   Baruch, S. *et al.* (2008) "Genetic Testing of Embryos: Practices and Perspectives of US *In Vitro* Fertilization Clinics."

31   Baruch, S. (2009) "Preimplantation Genetic Diagnosis and Parental Preferences: Beyond Deadly Disease."

32   Leigh, Suzanne. "Reproductive 'Tourism'" *USA Today – Health and Behavior*. USATODAY.com, May 2, 2005. Web. September 19. 2014. <http://usatoday30.usatoday.com/news/health/2005-05-02-reproductive-tourism_x.htm>.

33   Human Fertilisation and Embryology Bill. Bill 6, House of Lords. United Kingdom, 2007–2008.

34   NHS Commissioning Board Clinical Reference Group for Genetics. Clinical Commissioning Policy: Pre-Implantation Genetic Diagnosis (PGD). Rep. N.p.: NHS Commissioning Board, 2013.

35   Loi relative à la bioéthique. Loi no. 2011-814. French Parliament, 2011.

36   "The NHS in England." About the National Health Service (NHS) in England. NHS, n.d. Web. September 19, 2014.

37   Rodwin, Marc A. *Conflicts of Interest and the Future of Medicine: The United States, France, and Japan.* Oxford England: Oxford UP, 2011.

38   "Essential Health Benefits Standards: Ensuring Quality, Affordable Coverage." *– Centers for Medicare & Medicaid Services.* Centers for Medicare and Medicaid Services, February 20, 2013. Web. January 26, 2014. <http://www.cms.gov/CCIIO/Resources/Fact-Sheets-and-FAQs/ehb-2-20-2013.html>.

39   *Connecticut Medicaid: Summary of Services.* Medical Care Administration Department of Social Services, Connecticut Department of Social Services.

40   "State Laws Related to Insurance Coverage for Infertility Treatment." *Insurance Coverage for Infertility Laws.* National Conference of State Legislatures, June 2014. Web. September 19, 2014. <http://www.ncsl.org/issues-research/health/insurance-coverage-for-infertility-laws.aspx>.

41   Pers. comm. Dr Mark Hughes, Founder and Director of Genesis Genetics, January 15, 2014.

42   "The Costs of Infertility Treatment." *RESOLVE: The National Infertility Association.* RESOLVE, n.d. Web. September 19, 2014. <http://www.resolve.org/family-building-options/insurance_coverage/the-costs-of-infertility-treatment.html>.

DOI: 10.1057/9781137515445.0003

2
The Ethics of PGD and Its Relevance to Regulation

Abstract: *Taken together, Chapters 2 and 3 delve into the broad range of ethical issues surrounding the use of PGD. They are organized by broad questions such as "Should we be doing this at all?" and "What is a life worth living?" In Chapter 2, we discuss a number of general criticisms and defenses of the desire for control and choice that biotechnology generally and PGD in particular raise. We also begin to discuss a range of uses of PGD, including the avoidance of late onset genetic disease, positive selection for disabling conditions such as short stature or deafness, and sex selection. Relevant philosophical concepts and lines of ethical argument are discussed, such as the "expressivist" argument on selecting against a disability and the "non-identity problem" of harming an entity that would not otherwise exist if the putatively harmful action were not taken.*

Bayefsky, Michelle and Bruce Jennings. *Regulating Preimplantation Genetic Diagnosis in the United States: The Limits of Unlimited Selection.* New York: Palgrave Macmillan, 2015. DOI: 10.1057/9781137515445.0004.

DOI: 10.1057/9781137515445.0004

In this chapter, we address major ethical issues surrounding the different applications of PGD with a particular focus on how these ethical controversies relate to the governance and regulation of the use of PGD. We are not the first to identify these ethical questions, but our aim is to analyze which ethical concerns are (1) sufficiently well-grounded and (2) sufficiently relevant or practice-oriented to make a realistic contribution to the development of feasible and effective regulation.[1] By "well-grounded" we mean that the ethical and philosophical arguments appeal to ways of thinking and beliefs that are a part of reasonable public discourse in a pluralistic society. By "practice-oriented" we mean that there is a clear means of translating the concern into regulation, and that the concern is relevant given our current medical capabilities or advances that are likely to come about in the near future (such as whole-genome PGD).

This approach to the relationship between ethics and policy suggests the following stance. The governance of biotechnologies such as PGD does not need to be merely reactive or limited to a narrow conception of medical harm. There is a place for proactive or precautionary governance—law or regulation—but the justification and rationale for such precautionary governance should be based on reasonable ethical objection and reasonable questions concerning the legitimacy and public benefit of the technology. There need to be indications that society, medical practice, or the marketplace are in fact moving toward (starting to slide down the slippery slope, to use the most common metaphor) illegitimate applications of PGD. Such a movement can occur due to foreseeable growth of scientific knowledge and its technological momentum ("now that we can do something, we must do it").

The reasonable concerns about legitimacy and justification come from at least two areas. First, these concerns relate to the clinical, human, and social effects of developing technology. Second, they pertain to patterns of developing inequality of access to these technologies. The ethical discourse in policy governance involves both considerations of social justice as well as considerations of individual and social harm. For certain applications of PGD, some may believe that we have already completed the slide (for example, with regard to sex selection). For other potentially problematic applications, as we will discuss, there may be little reason to believe that such uses of PGD can or will ever be put into practice. Governance and regulation are never cost-free and their ethical justification must take goods and opportunities forgone, as well as harms and injustices forestalled, into consideration. Good arguments

DOI: 10.1057/9781137515445.0004

need to be made to justify devoting social and financial resources to the development and implementation of precautionary regulations.[2] It is also important to keep in mind that the ethical concerns raised in this chapter and the next must be carefully weighed against practical concerns and barriers to the regulation of PGD that will be addressed in Chapter 4.

The ethical critique of PGD: mastery and acceptance

The first and perhaps most open-ended question we raise is whether we should be using PGD at all; does using PGD overstep a moral boundary in our exertion of control over nature? Some argue that selecting some embryos over others via PGD is tinkering with nature or evolution in an unacceptable way. From a more religious perspective, the charge is that choosing some future children over others amounts to "playing God."

Some bioethicists, such as James Hughes, John Harris, and Julian Savulescu reject arguments based on claims that certain scientific or medical advances are "unnatural" or "ungodly" out of hand.[3] For example, Savulescu calls this type of argument "irrational" and feels no need to address its premises or implications. We agree that we would be ill-advised to accept the playing God critique without question and to ban the use of PGD outright on this basis alone. In fact, Baruch's public opinion data on the use of PGD indicate that only 19% of Americans surveyed believe that all uses of PGD should be banned.[4] Thus banning PGD altogether *solely* out of deference to the religious/ideological beliefs of a relatively small minority of Americans would amount to imposing that minority's religious/ideological views on the rest of society.[5]

Nevertheless, many people find it intuitively problematic for humans to exercise unlimited power over the world around us. In his book *The Case Against Perfection*, Michael Sandel articulates his unease with the "drive to mastery" suggested by the use of PGD.[6] He writes that we ought to "acknowledge the giftedness of life" and to do so by recognizing that "not everything in the world is open to any use we may desire or devise."[7] According to Sandel, humility is an essential virtue or feature of our "moral landscape," and some uses of PGD threaten to erode our humility in the face of nature, chance, or God.[8] He writes, "In a social world that prizes mastery and control, parenthood is a school for humility. That we care deeply about our children, and yet cannot choose the kind we want, teaches parents to be open to the unbidden.... The social

DOI: 10.1057/9781137515445.0004

basis of humility would also be diminished if people became accustomed to genetic self-improvement."[9] Sandel sees in America today an erosion of humility, together with two other virtues to which he takes it to be related: responsibility and solidarity. In that erosion of humanity, he sees social and cultural consequences that undermine personal happiness and the common good, and he also regrets the inherent loss of the sensibility and outlook contained within the notion of humility. He views humility as both an intrinsic and instrumental good.

Philosopher Frances Kamm criticizes Sandel's vagueness about the precise value of humility rather than mastery. For instance, Sandel writes that he is concerned that the desire for mastery will "leave us with nothing to affirm or behold outside our own will."[10] But Kamm points out that this claim is only valid if we view mastery as an end it itself rather than as a means to a further, hopefully good, end.[11] Furthermore, employing a kind of calculating moral reasoning that Sandel rejects, Kamm points out that even if mastery is pursued as an end in itself, other benefits that arise from mastery might outweigh this problematic motivation.[12]

Kamm may indeed have underscored a gap between the model of ethical reasoning Sandel uses and that more common in mainstream policy analysis. Mainstream analysis tends to keep a strict separation of means and ends, so that an attitude such as mastery is but a tool of producing other beneficial and justified social effects. In this separation, mastery will not transform the nature of the ends sought and can thus be contained and used with ethical safety. Or, if it should become an end in itself to some people, ethical justification can still be found in the value of what this attitude and purpose produce. Sandel, on the other hand, seems to see that means and ends interpenetrate and that certain orientations can crowd out and overwhelm other orientations. We can put mastery and humility on a balance sheet and see what good can be done using them, or we can see these as antagonists in a cultural struggle to maintain value pluralism and resist the dominance of any one orientation. The precision of Kamm's mode of argument contrasts with Sandel's, but it does not succeed in refuting Sandel's mode of argument on its own terms. The jury of history is still out—it remains to be seen whether biotechnology, genetic enhancement, and the like will ultimately be seen as mere tools of human purpose or as more active forces in shaping those purposes in substantive, and not necessarily humanistic, ways. We believe that it would be premature and imprudent to reject outright Sandel's fundamental claim—that there is something

DOI: 10.1057/9781137515445.0004

wrong with the drive to mastery and lack of humility that is embodied in and engendered by efforts to enhance children. That general concern, perhaps articulated in different ways, still needs to be taken seriously and warrants further investigation.

Sandel's argument that concerns about humility, responsibility, and solidarity should provide a basis for limiting or regulating the usage of PGD, at least for certain purposes, is within the realm of reasonable public debate and is an adequately grounded ethical perspective in that sense. It is not dependent upon a particular religious or cultural world-view, and if anything, is animated by an ethical pluralism and democratic public philosophy. To be sure, it reflects particular conceptions of how we ought to live our lives and approach the place of humans in the world. But these are conceptions that can be publicly understood, defended, and contested. They argue for limits on PGD in much the same spirit and in terms of some of the same values to which counter-arguments for the unrestricted use of PGD also appeal. Understood in this way, the range of values in arguments such as Sandel's—which are much broader than utilitarian concerns with preventing undue risk and harm of a rather directly medical or biological kind—should be admissible to the debate about whether and how to use PGD.

Admissibility does not in any way imply priority or dominance, however, and Sandel himself does not intend for his concerns about humility to trump all other considerations. He deliberately balances philosophical/spiritual considerations with practical considerations about personal and societal needs and does not find *all* uses of PGD to be morally problematic due to his concerns about humility and hubris. Sandel acknowledges that some uses of PGD may be justified and fall within the limits proscribed by humility whereas other uses remain problematic, though not necessarily impermissible.[13]

Sandel is vague about precisely what these limits are, but his general approach to the question "Should we be doing this at all?" is helpful. Yes, the use of PGD can be justified in certain situations, but we should be cautious and think carefully about our justifications for using PGD in those cases, and we ought to err on the side of inclusivity with regard to the arguments we will hear for and against various applications of PGD.

Sandel's approach to determining which uses of PGD are acceptable and unacceptable is also helpful. Sandel's acceptance of some uses over others rests on a distinction between healing and enhancing. By "healing," he means returning a person's physical state to "normal human

DOI: 10.1057/9781137515445.0004

functioning," though he does not attempt to define what normal human functioning is.[14] In the case of embryo selection, this would mean using PGD to ensure that a child does not have the kind of harmful genetic condition that would impede normal human functioning. Sandel accepts the use of PGD and other genetic technologies aimed at healing because he views health as an intrinsic good, one that is bounded and does not carry the risk of dragging parents into an "ever-escalating arms race."[15] People prefer good health to bad health, but a certain level of health is sufficient and there is no need for its unlimited maximization. Enhancing, by contrast, seems boundless. A child can always be better—stronger, faster, more beautiful, longer-living, or some preferable combination of ideal traits, whatever they may be. Pursuing these types of unlimited enhancements in children is what leads to a breakdown of humility, in Sandel's view, among other issues between parents and children to be discussed in the next section.

Sandel's distinction between healing and enhancing can be compared to the medical and nonmedical distinction made by insurance policies on PGD.[16] "Medical" would be akin to "healing" and "nonmedical" would include enhancing, as well as (debatably and circumstantially) value-neutral uses of PGD such as selection for eye color or sex. Beyond extreme examples, however, it is not obvious what should count as medical or nonmedical. Is selecting a child to serve as a tissue donor for a sick sibling a medical use of PGD? It is meant to heal *someone*, but not the child that is created via IVF and PGD. Is selecting against genes related to late-onset Alzheimer's a medical use of PGD? These are important questions with serious implications for what uses of PGD are appropriate based on Sandel's notion of humility.

Even if one does not subscribe to Sandel's views on the importance of humility, the healing–enhancing or related medical–nonmedical distinctions nonetheless carry weight because they comport well with well-accepted views on the goals of medicine. The Hippocratic Oath requires that doctors act for the "benefit of the sick"—in other words, to help those with medical conditions, or to heal.[17] The imperative to heal, which is commonly seen as the purpose of the medical profession,[18] does not mean that nonmedical uses of technology are morally impermissible. However, it does suggest that a doctor who uses technology in this manner is acting outside his or her role as a medical professional. Furthermore, given the risks of ovarian hyperstimulation associated with IVF and the unknown long-term risks that may be associated with

PGD, the requirement to heal and, concurrently, not to harm, indicates that doctors ought to think carefully before putting their patients at risk for the purpose of a nonmedical (or dubiously medical) procedure. The same issues can be raised about certain uses of plastic surgery, for example. We will not wade into the fascinating and complex debate about the purpose of medicine and the related moral restrictions and obligations of doctors. We seek only to demonstrate that while it is difficult to define terms such as "normal human functioning," "health," and "medical use of PGD," they remain relevant to the moral permissibility of certain applications of PGD.

In this section, we have discussed the issue of whether PGD should be used at all, based on conceptions of humility or the inherent need to limit humans' power over nature. We have concluded that these considerations ought not to be summarily dismissed, because humility can legitimately be considered as either an intrinsic or instrumental good, but that these kinds of arguments ought to be balanced against the need for certain uses of PGD. A strong case can be made for clearly beneficial, medical uses of PGD, and against harmful or unduly risky nonmedical uses. This distinction, while philosophically contentious, is attractive from a policy perspective for several reasons. As already mentioned, it fits well with traditional conceptions of the purpose of medicine, and is already built into the existing legal and regulatory framework for the governance of medical technology. Moreover, this distinction is used by the health insurance industry when deciding what applications of PGD to cover (to be discussed in Chapter 5). Finally, this distinction offers policymakers a stable, substantive, and ethically relevant means of characterizing different uses of PGD.

Parental duties and the genetic shaping of children

Another aspect of Sandel's discussion makes it a useful touchstone for considering the ethics of PGD—his argument concerning the potential impact of PGD on the parent–child relationship.[19] Sandel contends that parents who pay "large sums to select the sex of their child (for nonmedical reasons) or who aspire to bioengineer their child's intellectual endowments...are more likely to overreach, to express and entrench attitudes at odds with the norm of unconditional love." Parents should not value their children for the characteristics they possess or as "products of their

DOI: 10.1057/9781137515445.0004

will or instruments of their ambition"; they should value and love their children regardless.[20]

The norm of unconditional love

Sandel's argument about the potential breakdown of the parent–child relationship has been criticized for several reasons. First, while "unconditional love" is often used to express a seemingly boundless feeling of affection and protectiveness of parents toward their children, taken at face value, it is quite an extreme notion. Given examples of certain types of children, such as evil children, many people would find it understandable for parents not to love them, or even wrong for their parents to love them.[21] If one is willing to accept that in some cases parents need not love their children, why can't we accept parents who love their children in part because of particular qualities they have chosen for them? Moreover, if one is willing to accept that in some cases parents should attempt to change the personality and behavior of their children or should attempt to prevent or remove symptoms of disease, why preclude the mode of changing the traits and experiences of a future child represented by PGD?

Like Kamm's critique, however, these critical questions may miss the point of Sandel's argument. He does not aim to explain in a comprehensive, foolproof manner how all parents ought to feel toward all children. He is only pointing out that parents generally should love their children not for the qualities that they possess but because something about bringing a child into the world, and nurturing and raising that child, should generate feelings of love. The fact that to a certain extent parents *do* love children for their characteristics, as illustrated by the extreme example of parents not loving an evil child, does little to detract from the overall goal of Sandel's argument.

Where Sandel's argument is open to criticism is in its application of his views on ideal parent-to-child love to the case of genetic enhancement. He makes an implicit logical jump from "parents should generally love their children simply because they are their children" to "parents who try to select traits in their children love their children conditionally (and hence, insufficiently or improperly)." It is not at all clear, for example, that if parents attempted to select certain traits in their child and the selection process went awry, they would not love the resulting child just as much.[22]

Of course, there is no way to demonstrate empirically the relative quantities of love a parent would feel toward these two prospective

DOI: 10.1057/9781137515445.0004

children. However, a parallel may be drawn between the case of a poorly executed genetic selection procedure and cases in which women have tried and failed to obtain abortions. A 2013 study at the University of California, San Francisco, examined women who were turned away from abortion clinics with the aim of measuring the consequences of having to carry an unwanted pregnancy to term. Researchers found that only 5% of women wished they did not have the baby after it was born and the rest adjust and bond normally with the child.[23] If women come to adjust to the existence of originally unwanted children and grow to love these children similarly to how other women love always wanted children, it is plausible that people would end up loving a child without certain preferred characteristics just as much as a child who turned out exactly how they hoped. And if parents can love their children equally whether or not they possess certain preferred traits (within limits, e.g. excluding an evil child), then Sandel has not explained why parents who choose particular traits in their children must necessarily love their children insufficiently or improperly.

Over-the-top parenting attitudes

A portion of Sandel's analysis does not concern particular instances of parental love or attachment but rather general trends and orientations toward parenting as a social and cultural practice. He holds that genetic selection reinforces certain aspects of that practice, while undermining other methods of parenting. He takes issue with "overly ambitious" parents who get "carried away" and demand "all manner of accomplishments from their children," to the detriment of the child him or herself.[24] The main question is not, then, about love, but rather a style of parenting that Sandel finds problematic. Over-achieving helicopter parents (the kind who might pay $15,000 to have a child genetically enhanced) may still love their children very much, but nevertheless harm their children through this style of parenting and transmit poor values to future generations. This type of parenting, according to Sandel, will be encouraged in a society that allows and promotes the widespread use of PGD for enhancement purposes and that readily embraces new technological developments that will be forthcoming in this area.

Sandel's argument is paradoxical, however. On the one hand, he believes that our society and culture are already well along in the development of the styles and attitudes of parenting that he decries. But on the other hand, he views new biotechnological manipulations and enhancements

DOI: 10.1057/9781137515445.0004

as important causes of these same attitudes. Can it be shown that genetic selection adds something significant and additional to the actions of otherwise overzealous parents of already existing children? Parents can and do heavily influence their children's lives by the way in which they raise them, including by putting significant amounts of pressure on their children to succeed. Sandel clearly finds this problematic, but it is not clear why or in exactly what ways he thinks one more incremental biotechnology such as PGD will significantly exacerbate this cultural problem.

Dan Brock responds that incremental technological expansion can in fact lead to an incremental worsening of a cultural and moral climate. Brock's tone is less alarmed than Sandel's, but he is not complacent. He writes, "these new prospects for negative selection, positive selection, and genetic enhancement represent new, but hardly unprecedented, means of shaping future offspring and citizens; they are changes of degree and of means. Nevertheless, substantial changes of degree and means of this sort can raise new moral and policy issues, or make old issues more practically pressing."[25] Brock believes that we should be concerned about the development of selective genetic technology, but the exact nature of our concerns must be illuminated. With regard to degree, genetic selection is more permanent than the imprinting of values and cultural norms; a child cannot undo his or her genetic makeup,[26] whereas a child can, sometimes through radical rejection, sometimes through subtle reinterpretation, undo his or her upbringing. It is possible to appreciate the seriousness of deliberate preimplantation genetic manipulation, which is magnified because it involves heritable, intergenerational effects, without embracing genetic determinism, which has been overemphasized in popular culture,[27] and without denying that environmental factors contribute greatly to a person's health and behavior.[28] Moreover, while cultural continuity and tradition tend to be very strong in most historical periods, there is something even stronger about the inevitability of transmitting genetic characteristics from generation to generation. Thus, genetic technology does represent a significant difference in both the means and degree to which parents can exert influence on their children and future generations of our society.

Sandel takes it for granted that the controlling and perfecting instinct of parents who try to use PGD for enhancement purposes is problematic because he objects to the related method of parenting already existing children. His overall argument seems plausible, but his assumptions must be more clearly laid out.

DOI: 10.1057/9781137515445.0004

Selfishness and instrumentalization

Sandel hints at an accusation of selfishness in parents who attempt to engineer their children's qualities, as though they are doing it only for their own satisfaction. Susannah Baruch's classification of the different uses of PGD (mentioned in the previous chapter) into PGD for a serious heritable condition and PGD to satisfy parental preferences also alludes to this criticism, since the word "preferences" implies a certain level of frivolous self-centeredness in parents' decision making regarding their children.

However, we should not be too quick to judge the reasons behind parental desires to use PGD or to assume that parents are instrumentalizing their children for their own benefit. By endowing their child with certain genetic advantages, and by protecting them against certain genetic disadvantages, they may very well be attempting to act in the child's best interest. Furthermore, even if parents do aim to select certain characteristics that are specific to their preferences and intend to derive some benefit from their child's future success, it is generally considered acceptable that parents impart their own cultural traditions and values on their children and relish in their children's achievements. They may be treating their child as a means, but not a mere means.[29] The line between what parents want for themselves and for their children independently of themselves is often blurred because parents and children frequently have coinciding goals. We look favorably upon parents who work hard to help their children succeed and children who are grateful to their parents for their successes. Thus, except in extreme cases, where it is clear that what is best for the parent and child are distinct and the parent chooses the former, the selfishness critique cannot be a decisive condemnation of parents who use genetic selection to enhance their children.

Commodification

A second criticism implied by Sandel's comments on parental attitudes and genetic selection relates to the commodification of children. Imagine the scenario of a couple who enters a fertility specialist's office, takes out a checkbook, and says "Can I have a child with X, Y, and Z characteristics?" The transactional nature of the doctor–patient interaction seems problematic, as though by placing a monetary value on a child (and probably more money for children with "better" characteristics or more specifications), we are cheapening the value of that child's life. Or,

DOI: 10.1057/9781137515445.0004

perhaps more precisely, we are not so much lessening its value in quantitative terms as we are thinking about its value in the wrong way. We are thinking and talking about the "value" of a future human life as the outcome of an exchange transaction rather than locating it in a practice of care and beneficence that aims at the inherent value of a future life and its intrinsic moral worth.

However, the commodification objection can be (and has been) raised about all kinds of reproductive medical procedures, including IVF, gestational surrogacy, and compensated egg and sperm donation. All of these procedures, unless compensation is prohibited, involve paying money to receive a child. Thus unless we want to reject the use of all of these procedures, which would severely restrict the options of infertile couples, we cannot argue that the transaction itself is sufficient grounds for prohibiting the practice of medically assisted reproduction. We can, however, attempt to regulate the environment of using ART (including PGD) so that the experience of women and couples will not reinforce the sense of commodification or shape their attitudes toward their own choices or their new child in that way. Here the problem may not lie with PGD *per se*, but with the metaphors and meanings that our broader commercial and consumer culture imposes on it.

Parental control and the autonomy of the future child

In our view, there are two primary issues illustrated by the scenario presented earlier. The first is that the parents seem to be insufficiently respectful of the creation of a new life. In comparison to the significance of a new person coming into being, their requests for this or that characteristic seem frivolous. This is essentially Sandel's humility critique. Though intuitively compelling, this critique cannot serve as the *sole* justification for prohibiting certain applications of PGD because doing so would require imposing one view of the types of beliefs/ideas that people ought to value on all of society.[30] The second issue lies in the degree of control that the parents in the scenario earlier are exerting over their future child by choosing its specific characteristics. While some take issue with parents using PGD for nonmedical reasons and selecting for characteristics in their child that have nothing to do with health, it seems even worse for parents to choose multiple characteristics aimed at enhancing their child or satisfying the parents' own cultural preferences or ideals, or to enter the doctor's office with a laundry list of requests. Here the popular term, "designer babies," seems apt. Specifying

DOI: 10.1057/9781137515445.0004

multiple characteristics indicates that parents aim to exert more and more control over their future child's qualities. We have argued that the control afforded by genetic selection is distinct in means and degree from that which stems from the way a child is raised,[31] but it remains to be explained what precisely is wrong with parents exerting this kind of control over their children, aside from a potential issue with the parenting style that will likely be practiced by such parents once the child is born.[32]

The control exerted over a child by choosing his or her characteristics can be considered problematic from the standpoint of that child's autonomy. Joel Feinberg's "right to an open future" argument regarding mandatory education, later applied to genetic selection by Dena Davis, asserts that children possess "rights in trust" that, while not exercised until adulthood, ought nevertheless be protected.[33] To illustrate this concept, Davis offers the example of the right to reproduce. Although a young child cannot physically exercise the right to reproduce, and a teenager may lack the resources or other means of exercising that right, children should nevertheless not be sterilized because sterilization would preclude the ability to exercise the right to reproduce upon reaching adulthood. The basic point is that respecting a child's autonomy requires that choices not be made on behalf of a child in such a way that "narrows the scope of her choices when she grows up."[34]

The difficulty with the open future argument is that it seems to rely on empirical generalizations about what actions will or will not restrict a child's future. Such generalizations may become inaccurate over time due to social or technological changes, and they are difficult to apply to the circumstances of an individual child. Moreover, it is difficult, if not impossible, to quantify the number of options children with different genetic traits will have open to them.[35] Beyond obviously restrictive and rather extreme actions to change the future life of a child, such as sterilization (and potentially selecting for a disability, which will be discussed later in this chapter), the open future argument thus does not provide much specific guidance or justification for limiting parental behavior or selection of genetic characteristics in their children. If anything, this argument may justify parental choices to use PGD in order to select for genetically enhanced children, who then would presumably have more future options open to them if they were very intelligent, talented, or attractive.

In order to provide guidance for the ethical uses of PGD, then, the concept of an open future requires an explicit normative account of what

DOI: 10.1057/9781137515445.0004

"open" means and what the child's future should be open to. Arguing that a reproductive decision based on PGD will be justified if it gives the child more choices, and not justified if it gives the child fewer choices, is not sufficient. What, then, might be the basis for arguing that nonmedical uses of PGD for the selection of certain traits violates the future child's autonomy? This question is complicated by the fact that children never get to choose their own genetic characteristics; if their parents do not choose them for them, then the randomness or chance involved in the fertilization of an egg by a particular sperm or the implantation of one embryo over another determines children's genes. Nevertheless, the notion of autonomy does not only imply the ability to make choices for oneself, it also implies freedom from others making choices on one's behalf.[36] Thus, it is precisely *because* parents are the ones deciding the genetic characteristics of their children, rather than chance (or God), that the child's autonomy is restricted. While parents make all kinds of decisions on behalf of their children, we have contended that there is a difference in degree and means involved with genetic selection, which makes this exercise of parental control particularly autonomy-restricting.

We conclude, therefore, that certain uses of PGD should be limited in order to protect the child's future autonomy, and that this limitation would be consistent with desirable patterns of value and action both at the level of private parental decision making and at the social and cultural level. Respecting the autonomy rights of the future child and the value of open parenting creates ethical obligations that have a bearing on the decisions of parents, and perhaps on the decisions of individual physicians and other health professionals as well. But are these consid-erations a sufficient basis for restricting the uses of PGD as a matter of law and public policy? In Chapter 4, we will examine whether it might be reasonable to institute regulations in order to protect rights of future children and to mitigate certain parental and cultural attitudes. At the very least, these are relevant considerations that should be factored into the public regulation of PGD.

The ethical case for PGD: procreative beneficence

Having considered various critiques of the project of genetically shaping children through the use of PGD, we turn now to the positive ethical

DOI: 10.1057/9781137515445.0004

case for doing so. Notable here is the work of Savulescu, who views the prospect of creating so-called designer babies as an ethical opportunity that we have an obligation to pursue. He argues that in order to provide the best life possible to future children, we are morally obligated to use the means provided by PGD to ensure that children are both free from genetic disease and possess the nonmedical genetic characteristics that make them most likely to lead the best possible life.[37] He calls this principle "Procreative Beneficence," and bases his arguments on the standard utilitarian concept of maximizing overall well-being. The moral obligation of parents to use PGD is thus limited by what applications would actually detract from overall well-being. For example, large-scale sex selection for males over females would likely reduce overall well-being in the long term, but sex selection on a smaller scale, if it made the resulting children somehow better-off, would not only be recommended but also morally obligatory.[38]

We have already discussed our objection to Savulescu's dismissal of concerns related to humility in shaping future children, which is apparent in his encouragement of the use of PGD whenever a child's well-being might be improved. While Sandel views humility and accepting the givenness, or giftedness, of a child whose genes you have not chosen as an important aspect of parenting, Savulescu seems to view choosing the genes of one's children as an extension of rational risk avoidance in parenting made possible by advances in science and technology, the way that others might view abstaining from alcohol while pregnant, for example.[39] Interestingly, both Sandel and Savulescu reject the notion that prospective parents have no moral obligations to beings that do not yet exist, but their respective understandings of what those obligations are differ diametrically. Savulescu takes a rather straightforward utilitarian approach in developing his "Procreative Beneficence" principle. His work illustrates some difficulties that utilitarian ethical theory encounters in dealing with PGD.

First, Savulescu does not consider autonomy-based arguments for limiting the use of PGD for nonmedical reasons. Utilitarians are often criticized for insufficiently valuing individual rights, including autonomy, in the process of maximizing overall well-being. Savulescu is vulnerable to this criticism. He ideally would like to maximize the well-being of each child in order to maximize overall well-being, but he does not care if well-being is maximized at the expense of the future children's rights. Moreover, the ideal of well-being itself is complex in

DOI: 10.1057/9781137515445.0004

the context of the types of traits and conditions related to the genetic shaping of future children through PGD. Here it is especially difficult, if not impossible, to define and measure well-being, and it is very difficult to predict what genetic modifications—among the nonmedical uses of PGD, at least—will result in the greatest overall well-being. While studies can be done about whether blond, tall, and athletic people tend to be happier than short, un-athletic, brown-haired people, such studies would have many confounding factors relating to class and race and it is not at all clear that they would continue to hold true if selection became commonplace and widespread.

A final objection to the Procreative Beneficence principle regards equitable access to PGD and the long-term effects of this technology on the condition of overall social inequality. In the future, will one's social achievements and relative success reflect competitive merit or will they reflect the work of genetic enhancement that one's parents could afford? If genetic science ever reaches the point where we can select for or against complex multigene traits, and access to such interventions is limited only to the most well off, then the inequity of the chance to increase their child's likelihood of having the best possible life will be a serious social injustice. Like other utilitarian theorists, Savulescu is interested in increasing aggregate net well-being across the population as a whole; he is not concerned if an optimal outcome is achieved via a distributional pattern of social resources that is highly inequitable.[40] Indeed, he explicitly maintains that we should obey his principle "even if this maintains or increases social inequality."[41] From a rights-based or "deontological" ethical perspective, using PGD for enhancement purposes without providing a means of equalizing access, such as public funding, would be unjust and unfair. However, obtaining public funding for PGD for enhancement purposes is extremely unrealistic considering that the United States does not have a single-payer system and insurance coverage for fertility services is very limited.

Savulescu takes the extreme position that PGD is morally obligatory even for nonmedical purposes, but others limit their claims regarding moral obligations to medical uses of PGD. Malek and Daar make the case that there is an ethical duty to use PGD when parents know their offspring "is at substantial risk of inheriting a serious genetic condition" and that there might even be a legal duty to perform PGD when a couple is already using IVF and knows that any future children are at a substantial risk of having a serious genetic condition.[42] Malek and Daar

DOI: 10.1057/9781137515445.0004

do not argue from a purely utilitarian point of view; they also consider the number of options open to the future child and whether there is any injustice in having to suffer from a serious genetic condition that could have been avoided.

It is significant that Malek and Daar base their argument on a paradigmatic case—using PGD to select against autosomal recessive polycystic kidney disease (ARPKD). ARPKD is paradigmatic because it is a very severe disorder; many infants with ARPKD do not survive their first year, and those who survive suffer from organ failure and numerous additional serious complications. Malek and Daar are notably vague, however, about what other cases might warrant a legal (and ethical) obligation for performing PGD.[43] The question of what constitutes a serious or severe disease is a very difficult but relevant question, both when trying to determine personal moral duties for parents and physicians and when trying to determine ethically appropriate public policy and regulations. It does not make sense to argue for moral or legal obligations, or to design regulations for permissible uses of PGD, without clarifying what we mean by "serious disease" and how far our obligations extend. If there are moral gray areas (e.g. regarding selection against a disability such as deafness), it is difficult to claim that there is a moral or legal duty to use PGD. Similarly, it is difficult to prohibit certain uses of PGD in this area of moral uncertainty. How regulations can be designed to deal with moral gray zones will be discussed in the next chapter.

Beyond the medical and scientific limitations of PGD in the present and foreseeable future, the creation of designer babies presents a sad vision of the journey of becoming a parent. In practice, genetic selection would involve creating as many embryos as possible, testing all of them genetically, and picking the embryo with the fewest mutations.[44] Parents would likely choose to select against harmful conditions before they would select for positive traits, especially relatively superficial ones such as eye color. Thus rather than designing a child according to their preferences, parents would have to satisfy themselves with selecting the least mutated embryo, and to live with the knowledge of the mutations carried by the chosen embryo. Selecting the best of a group of embryos, all of which possess at least some unfavorable mutations, is hardly a happy way for a life to begin or for people to embark on the journey of having a child. Taken alone, this concern with permitting PGD for a wide range of conditions would not justify restricting the use of PGD, but it could serve as a reality check for those who view the prospect of creating designer children favorably.

DOI: 10.1057/9781137515445.0004

Notes

1   See, for example: Wilkinson, Stephen. *Choosing Tomorrow's Children: The Ethics of Selective Reproduction.* Oxford, England: Clarendon, 2010; Scott, Rosamund. *Choosing between Possible Lives.* Oxford: Hart, 2007.

2   Robertson, John. "Assisting Reproduction, Choosing Genes and the Scope of Reproductive Autonomy."" *The George Washington Law Review* 76.6 (2008): 1490–1513.

3   Savulescu, Julian. "Procreative Beneficence: Why We Should Select the Best Children." *Bioethics* 15.5–6 (2001): 413–426. Hughes, James. *Citizen Cyborg: Why Democratic Societies Must Respond to the Redesigned Human of the Future.* Cambridge, MA: Westview, 2004. Harris, John. *Enhancing Evolution: The Ethical Case for Making Better People.* Princeton, NJ: Princeton UP, 2007. We will focus on Savulescu's views in this section because they are neatly presented, directly relevant to genetic selection, and in many ways representative of prominent ideas in the secular bioethics community. Savulescu's ideas on procreative autonomy, which will be discussed later, do represent an extreme pro-enhancement position. However, the comparison of Savulescu's and Sandel's views is meant to illustrate the spectrum from liberal to conservative views on the use of technology such as PGD for genetic enhancement purposes.

4   Baruch, Susannah. "PGD: Genetic Testing of Embryos in the United States." *JRC European Commission.* Johns Hopkins University, February 15, 2009. Web. January 26, 2014.

5   There may be other reasons to formulate laws based on the views of a minority of Americans and it can sometimes be appropriate to create laws for reasons that stem from religious or ideological views. However, religious/ ideological views alone should not dictate practice in a country that values democracy and the separation of church and state.

6   Sandel, Michael J. *The Case against Perfection: Ethics in the Age of Genetic Engineering.* Cambridge, MA: Belknap of Harvard UP, 2007. Page 27.

7   Ibid.

8   Ibid. Page 87.

9   Ibid. Page 86.

10 Sandel, Michael J. "The case against perfection." *Atlantic Monthly* 293(3): 51–62.

11 Kamm, F. M. *Bioethical Prescriptions to Create, End, Choose, and Improve Lives.* Oxford: Oxford UP, 2013. Page 328.

12 Ibid. Page 330.

13 Kamm repeatedly criticizes Sandel for leaping from the assertion that certain motivations and attitudes are problematic to the claim that certain actions ought to be impermissible (*Bioethical Prescriptions,* pages 328–331). But Sandel does not directly state that X, Y, and Z actions ought to be impermissible

DOI: 10.1057/9781137515445.0004

because of the attitudes that they embody and engender—perhaps unsatisfyingly, he aims to describe the problematic desires, beliefs, and characters that both cause and are created by a lack of humility and stops short of precisely delineating permissible action. Thus not only does he allow for non-humility considerations to outweigh humility considerations at times, he also does not claim that all morally problematic uses of PGD ought to be banned on the basis of the humility argument alone.

14   Ibid. Page 47.

15   Ibid. Page 49.

16   See, for example: "GENE.00002 Preimplantation Genetic Diagnosis Testing." *GENE.00002 Preimplantation Genetic Diagnosis Testing.* Anthem, Inc., October 8, 2013. Web. March 29, 2014. <http://www.anthem.com/medicalpolicies/policies/mp_pw_a049872.htm>.

17   Hippocrates. "The Hippocratic Oath." *Greek Medicine.* Trans. Michael North. U.S. National Library of Medicine, July 2, 2012. Web. February 13, 2014. <https://www.nlm.nih.gov/hmd/greek/greek_oath.html>.

18   Egnew, Thomas. "The Meaning of Healing: Transcending Suffering." *Annals of Family Medicine* 3.3 (2005): 255–262.

19   See also Thomas Murray's discussion of "Perfectibilism and Parenthood," in *The Worth of a Child.* Berkeley: University of California Press, 1996. Pages 131–137.

20   Sandel, Michael J. *The Case against Perfection: Ethics in the Age of Genetic Engineering.* Page 49.

21   Wilkinson, Stephen. *Choosing Tomorrow's Children: The Ethics of Selective Reproduction.* Page 24.

22   Ibid. Page 29.

23   Lang, Joshua. "What Happens to Women Who Are Denied Abortions?" *The New York Times*, June 12, 2013. Web. February 22, 2014.

24   Sandel, Michael J. *The Case against Perfection: Ethics in the Age of Genetic Engineering.* Page 50.

25   Brock, Dan W. "Shaping Future Children: Parental Rights and Societal Interests." *Journal of Political Philosophy* 13.4 (2005): 377–398.

26   Gene editing is an emerging line of research in genetics, but changing the genes in all the cells of a person's body is not a realistic option, at least for the foreseeable future.

27   See, for example, the opening scene in the 1997 movie *Gattaca*, in which the protagonist's entire future is foretold from the output of a genetic sequencing machine.

28   Buchanan, Allen E., Dan W. Brock, Norman Daniels, and Daniel Wikler. *From Chance to Choice: Genetics and Justice.* Cambridge, U.K.: Cambridge UP, 2000. Page 23.

DOI: 10.1057/9781137515445.0004

29   Wilkinson, Stephen. *Choosing Tomorrow's Children: The Ethics of Selective Reproduction*. Page 134.

30   Although sometimes it may be appropriate to create laws or regulations in response to serious moral objections to a certain practice (e.g. the 13th Amendment), in this case the fundamental question is not one of inequality or basic human rights, but rather a judgment about what values individuals should hold dear. The issue of when and why "moral legislation" is sometimes acceptable is a complicated question that we cannot fully address here, but we submit that regulating PGD on the basis of the humility objection alone would take moral legislation too far. This is at least in part because the societal-level (vs. individual-level) effects of valuing humility are not, in our view, sufficiently immediate to warrant government intervention.

31   It is not necessarily true that using genetic selection to select certain traits in a child is more controlling than the manner in which one raises a child, depending on what qualities we are comparing. For example, selecting a child with blue eyes will likely have a less significant effect on a child's life than deciding to train that child from age two to become a star athlete. However, when comparing similar qualities, like selecting for strength, speed, and height versus raising a child to be a star basketball player, the impact of genetic selection seems greater because it is physically ingrained and irreversible.

32   Sandel does not clearly distinguish between parents' attitude toward selecting children with certain traits and parent's attitude toward child-rearing once the children have been born. He seems to be primarily concerned with the likelihood that parents who exhibit controlling and perfecting behavior during selection will be similarly controlling and perfecting once the child is born, but he does not address the notion that parental obligations and attitudes toward prospective children might be different from those toward existing children.

33   Feinberg, Joel. "The Child's Right to an Open Future." *Whose Child? Children's Rights, Parental Authority, and State Power*. Totowa, New Jersey: Littlefield, Adams &, 1980. 124–153; Davis, Dena. "Genetic Dilemmas and the Child's Right to an Open Future." *The Hastings Center Report* 27.2 (1997): 7–15.

34   Ibid.

35   Wilkinson, Stephen. *Choosing Tomorrow's Children: The Ethics of Selective Reproduction*. Page 47.

36   Fallon, Jr Richard H. "Two Senses of Autonomy." *Stanford Law Review* 46.4 (1994): 875–905; Christman, John. "Autonomy in Moral and Political Philosophy." *Stanford Encyclopedia of Philosophy*. Stanford University, July 28, 2003. Web. February 21, 2014.

37   Savulescu, Julian. (2001) "Procreative Beneficence: Why We Should Select the Best Children."

DOI: 10.1057/9781137515445.0004

38   Ibid.

39   Of course, a pregnant woman may abstain from drinking alcohol in order
to avoid *harming* an already existing being, whereas it is difficult to argue
that by not selecting for the best possible genes we are harming a being
that not would have existed otherwise. This is the nonidentity problem,
which Savulescu skirts by focusing on overall well-being rather than harm.
Nevertheless, it is interesting to note that he seems to expect that prospective
parents act like actual parents when making decisions regarding their future
child.

40   If a pattern of unequal distribution produces such a widespread negative
effect on the well-being of the least well off that it drags down the overall
population happiness to a suboptimal state, then a utilitarian approach
would seek an alternative means to achieve an aggregate net benefit, perhaps
by designing equalizing measures to counteract relative deprivation within
the population. But here equality and various kinds of moral protections
for individuals, such as rights, are means to an aggregate end; they are not
morally significant in and of themselves.

41   Savulescu, Julian. (2001) "Procreative Beneficence: Why We Should Select
the Best Children."

42   Malek, Janet, and Judith Daar. "The Case for a Parental Duty to Use
Preimplantation Genetic Diagnosis for Medical Benefit." *The American
Journal of Bioethics* 12.4 (2012): 3–11.

43   Francis, Leslie Pickering, and Anita Silvers. "A Wrongful Case for Parental
Tort Liability." *The American Journal of Bioethics* 12.4 (2012): 15–17.

44   Pers. comm. Dr Mark Hughes, Founder and Director of Genesis Genetics,
January 15, 2014.

3

Drawing Ethical Lines

Abstract: *In this chapter, we discuss the different ethical views regarding the various options for the use of PGD to select among embryos for implantation, gestation, and birth. In particular, we address the notions of parental autonomy and reproductive rights as they apply to PGD. As the differing ethical problems are presented, they are evaluated for their relative strength and relevance to the question of whether PGD should be regulated in the United States in the near future. Arguments are considered less compelling if they are predicated on unrealistic scientific predictions, ignore political/social circumstances in the United States, or would create undesirable consequences if taken to their logical ends.*

Bayefsky, Michelle and Bruce Jennings. *Regulating Preimplantation Genetic Diagnosis in the United States: The Limits of Unlimited Selection.* New York: Palgrave Macmillan, 2015. DOI: 10.1057/9781137515445.0005.

Thus far, our analysis of the impact of PGD on parent–child relations has involved a discussion of parental attempts to choose one or more nonmedical characteristics in children. However, it is important to remember that the current limitations of genetic technology, reproductive medicine, and embryology are such that it is not possible for couples to select for multiple genes in a future child without undergoing numerous IVF cycles and incurring tens, if not hundreds of thousands of dollars in costs. Even so, the limited number of healthy embryos would not allow parents to truly design their children. Applying the ethical concerns laid out in the previous chapter to the issue of regulation requires that we be realistic about what is practically feasible, not just what is theoretically possible, and the prospect of designer babies does not appear to be a realistic concern. Nonetheless, the conclusions we have reached about parental attitudes and control also apply to applications of PGD that are available at present, such as HLA matching to save an older child, selection against adult onset disease, nonmedical sex selection, and selection for a disability. These applications will be addressed in greater depth in the present chapter.

Defining disease

Many arguments about acceptable and unacceptable uses of PGD are predicated on the notion that a line can be drawn, if not precisely then roughly, between medical and nonmedical uses of PGD, since the medical uses seem *prima facie* more appropriate for a "medical" technology and since the prevention of harm and suffering involved in these uses of PGD is ethically compelling. And the very notion of a "medical" use of PGD depends on our definition of disease. There are three main ways to view the relevance of disease to the use of PGD: (1) the detection of a genetic condition likely to cause disease is irrelevant to whether or not PGD should be used, (2) PGD should be used to select against only conditions that we determine to be a disease, and (3) PGD should only be used to select against *severe* or *serious* diseases. Savulescu's views fall into the first category; he writes that "It is not disease which is important but its impact on well-being." Malek and Daar use the third category to define when the use of PGD is morally obligatory (i.e. for severe diseases). Sandel might question whether PGD is ever morally *obligatory*, but he would appeal to the third category to define what uses are morally

DOI: 10.1057/9781137515445.0005

permissible. Others who support selection against disabilities such as deafness, certain adult onset diseases such as late onset Alzheimer's, or genes that indicate a higher risk for getting a disease, such as the BRCA breast cancer genes, may agree with the view expressed in the second category if they believe that these are not severe diseases that nonetheless warrant negative selection. Clearly, the concept of a "disease" (sometimes used broadly enough to encompass the notion of "disability") is contested and ambiguous, but it seems indispensible to the project of drawing lines in ethics and public policy on the subject of PGD.

In 2013, the American Medical Association decided to classify obesity as a disease, against the recommendations of a committee that had investigated and written a report on the subject.[1] The report noted that there was no "single, clear, authoritative, and widely-accepted definition of disease,"[2] but delegates decided that the potential public health benefits of classification outweighed the drawbacks, including the definitional concern. When weighing the pros and cons of classification, the committee considered several definitions of disease. The first was that all three of the following criteria must be met: (1) an impairment of the normal functioning of some aspect of the body, (2) characteristic signs or symptoms and (3) resultant harm or morbidity to the entity affected.[3] Another definition was based on biostatistical theory: "Deviation from species-typical functioning...deviation from the average." A third included causative agents: "An impairment of the normal state of the living animal...or one of its parts that interrupts or modifies the performance of the vital functions, is typically manifested by distinguishing signs and symptoms, and is a response to environmental factors...specific causative agents...inherent defects of the organism (as genetic anomalies), or to a combination of these factors."[4] All of these definitions of disease are broad and rely on our being able to ascertain what is "normal." The statistical definition is appealing because it provides a concrete method for defining "normal," but it is so broad that it includes any genetic anomaly that may or may not cause disease-like symptoms. The other definitions seem more relevant to what we think of as disease, but do not provide a clear, seemingly objective way of defining "normal functioning" or "normal state."

A definition of disease can never be entirely objective or universalizable, however. The AMA report noted that the medical community's definition of disease has always been "heavily influenced by contexts of time, place and culture as much as scientific understanding of disease

DOI: 10.1057/9781137515445.0005

processes."⁵ The ultimate decision of the AMA to classify obesity as a disease is indicative of the culture and context-specific nature of our definition of disease. By extension, decisions regarding the allowance of PGD for selection against certain conditions are highly contingent upon our current understanding and perception of the diseases caused by the genetic anomalies.

It is noteworthy that the first definition of disease cited earlier requires that the condition cause harm or morbidity, unlike the other definitions, which merely require that something be atypical about the functioning of the affected organism. "Harm" is a vague term with varying degrees, but it also accurately describes what most people assume about disease: that the disease negatively impacts the person with the condition. If the disease did not have a negative impact on the life of the affected person, its relevance to the use of PGD would be limited. Serious discussion of PGD occurs when it is intended to prevent harm or produce benefit, especially when it can preclude giving birth to a child with a disease that does substantial harm to the affected person, their family, and potentially society as a whole.

It could be argued that by not using PGD when certain genetic deviations are suspected, we either deliberately or inadvertently produce disease or disability to which society must then respond. That may be ethically wrong; in any case it is very expensive. For example, could some of the problems now discovered by newborn screening be prevented by PGD? If we consider societal harm in our calculation of whether or not to allow PGD, negative selection against these diseases may be warranted.

If we use the first definition of disease offered by the AMA report on obesity, and consider harm to the affected individual, the family, and society at large, the use of PGD would theoretically be warranted in many cases. However, we cannot neglect to weigh the negative impact of undergoing IVF and PGD due to the associated physical discomfort, risk to the woman, and significant expense. The question becomes, then, *how much* harm must the disease cause to the affected person in order to outweigh the physical and financial costs of carrying out PGD? The second approach to the relevance of defining disease for performing PGD implies that whenever the harm that the disease will cause the future child is greater than the burden of performing IVF and PGD on the parents, family, and society, PGD may ethically be performed.

By contrast, the third approach, that PGD should only be performed in order to prevent severe or serious diseases, introduces considerations other than direct harm and burden to the affected parties. This approach

DOI: 10.1057/9781137515445.0005

carries with it an assumption that PGD is generally not appropriate, for example due to concerns about humility, autonomy, eugenics, or the effect of negative selection on existing populations with the condition (the latter two concerns will be discussed in greater depth later in this chapter and in the next chapter). An exception may be made, however, in order to prevent the resulting child from having a severe or serious disease. In other words, a disease must cause a significant amount of harm to the future child in order to balance out all harm-related and other reasons for avoiding the use of PGD.

The writings of many individual analysts, as well as many organizational position statements and guidelines, rely on the notion that a significant amount of harm must be caused by a disease in order to warrant negative genetic selection. For example, the ASRM practice guidelines on PGD published in 2008 say that IVF with PGD "represents a major scientific advance" for "couples known to be at risk for having children with a heritable and debilitating genetic disease." "Debilitating" implies a great deal of harm, but the ASRM guidelines also say that "PGD is indicated for couples at risk for transmitting a specific genetic disease or abnormality to their offspring."[6] The guidelines seem to vacillate between the second and third approaches to using PGD—can PGD be used for any disease, or only debilitating diseases? A 2004 report by the President's Council on Bioethics writes that PGD "enables parents to avoid the deep grief and hardship that accompany the birth of a child with dreaded and incurable diseases such as cystic fibrosis and Tay Sachs."[7] Another report by President Bush's Bioethics Council (on which Michael Sandel served as a member) attempts to distinguish between healing and enhancing by citing the goal of PGD as creating "healthier children...who are better only in the sense of being free of severe disease and deformity."[8] The report explains our desire to use PGD in the following manner:

> People welcome these technologies for multiple reasons: compassion for the suffering of those afflicted with genetic diseases; the wish to spare families the tragedy and burden of caring for children with deadly and devastating illnesses; sympathy for those couples who might otherwise forego having children, for fear of passing on heritable disorders; an interest in reducing the economic and social costs of caring for the incurable; and hopes for progress in the overall health and fitness of human society.[9]

Words like "devastating," "tragedy," and "dreaded" indicate that a high degree of harm must come to the individual, family, or society in order for the use of PGD to be justified.

DOI: 10.1057/9781137515445.0005

These documents also suggest that PGD is most appropriate when used to prevent the birth of children with incurable diseases that cause premature death—a more stringent standard than "serious" or "severe" disease. Breast cancer may not meet this standard, given the availability of preventative measures such as genetic screening and prophylactic mastectomy. Selection against certain disabilities, such as deafness, would also not be considered appropriate uses of PGD according to these President's Council documents.[10]

When we begin to use PGD for certain designated conditions that can be effectively treated or managed, but not for all conditions that are species-atypical and cause some measure of harm, then we enter a medical and moral gray area and must be wary of making ethically arbitrary distinctions. Words like "serious" or "severe," which are very difficult to define, may begin to seem appealing precisely because of their vagueness, which allows for flexibility in determining when PGD is appropriate. What is considered to be a serious condition is very personal and subjective because it depends on a person and their family's ability to cope with the condition, not only on the nature of the disease and its symptoms.[11] Some believe that flexibility in the conditions for which PGD may be used is desirable because parents should be able to determine for themselves whether a condition is sufficiently serious.[12] Others believe that parents should be afforded a degree of flexibility, but within certain limits; not just any condition can be deemed "serious" or "not serious" by a parent. The use of terms such as "serious" and "severe" indicate that while precise lines cannot be easily drawn between appropriate and inappropriate disease-related applications of PGD, perhaps we should be on guard against the tendency to expand the scope of utilization of a technology over time, and we should think carefully about the counseling that parents receive prior to a decision to use PGD. We should strive to avoid the ethical errors of overutilization of a technology like PGD, even if it is paid for out of pocket by affluent prospective parents, in addition to the ethical errors of underutilization and unfair access.

Selecting against deafness

Deafness is often used as a paradigmatic example of a condition for which there is disagreement regarding its seriousness and subsequently whether PGD should be used to select for or against it. It is generally

DOI: 10.1057/9781137515445.0005

considered to be a disability, which, like disease, can be understood in different ways. Rosamund Scott has written extensively on ethical and legal issues related to PGD and pre-natal diagnosis and defines disability as "a condition or impairment [which] may result in physical pain or psychological suffering but will not necessarily do so, contrary to some presumptions."[13] Her definition takes into account the fact that many deaf people, for example, do not consider themselves to be *suffering* from deafness—it is simply a hearing impairment to which they have managed to adjust.

Others do not consider deafness to be a negative variation at all. University of Connecticut Professor Laura Mauldin, who attended Gallaudet University as a hearing person, believes that deafness is simply "a neutral variation in human bodies."[14] As such, if regulators were to restrict the use of PGD to medical purposes, she does not feel that testing for deafness should be permitted, though as a feminist, she also believes women should have the freedom to make such reproductive choices.[15] Mauldin realizes that the perception of deafness as a neutral variation is a minority view, though. While it is certainly a positive development that some deaf people have been able to adjust to their condition to the extent that they do not feel disadvantaged, there is a danger of overly romanticizing such an impairment or discussing only what can be gained through it but not what may be lost or precluded. Deafness is an impairment of one of the major senses, and would be considered a disability under Scott's definition. Similarly, the American with Disabilities Act defines disability as "(A) a physical or mental impairment that substantially limits one or more major life activities of such individual; (B) a record of such an impairment; or (C) being regarded as having such an impairment."[16] Even if deafness does not substantially limit major life activities for some deaf people, the condition would nonetheless be considered a disability under (C)—because other people commonly view deafness as a disability.

Mauldin's objection to selection against deafness could be modified to the assertion that deafness is not a sufficiently *serious* condition to warrant negative selection via PGD. Others, such as Dena Davis, disagree and claim that deafness does negatively impact people living with the disability and substantially limits major life activities.[17] Researchers have also demonstrated that families with hearing-impaired children are more likely to have poorer health statuses and to live below the poverty level[18] and that deafness correlates with lower income and education levels,

DOI: 10.1057/9781137515445.0005

as well as higher unemployment.[19] As noted previously, however, some judgments about the severity of a condition may depend on the ability of the affected person and his or her family to adapt. This means that the negative impact of deafness on children will depend on whether they and their families can cope emotionally and financially with the disability.[20] But we would not be comfortable saying that parents with fewer means should feel more compelled to select against deafness than parents who can afford to provide a deaf child with good educational opportunities and a supportive environment. Thus although some people and families will not view deafness as a serious disability, we cannot prohibit selection against deafness on this basis.

Even if we assume that deafness is a serious disability, some still believe that we should not use PGD to select against it because it sends a negative message to and about existing deaf people. This is called the "expressivist" argument against using pre-natal or preimplantation genetic tests to select against certain conditions.[21] Savulescu does not find the expressivist argument persuasive; he writes that selecting against a disability "does not necessarily imply that the lives of those who now live with disability are less deserving of respect and are less valuable." He further notes that it "is important to distinguish between disability and persons with disability" and asserts that "Selection reduces the former, but is silent on the value of the latter."[22]

Yet, the expressivist concern should not be quickly dismissed.[23] Savulescu's distinction between a disability and people with that disability only holds so long as deaf people view themselves as distinct from their condition. While it seems plausible that a deaf person's core identity or self-perceived essence is not dependent on his or her disability, it is nonetheless difficult to assume that having a disability is entirely separate from one's identity. Therefore, it is understandable that deaf people may view selection against future deaf children as a statement that is relevant to themselves. As Savulescu notes, however, selecting against deafness is not an indication that existing deaf people are less deserving of respect or that the life of a deaf person is worth less than the life of a hearing person.[24] It is simply a comment that we generally consider it better to live without deafness than with deafness. This is a claim that is controversial for Deaf Pride advocates such as Mauldin, of course. Moreover, despite Savulescu's logic, it is still understandable that persons living with disabilities—in a society that tends to treat them inequitably and provide inadequate medical and social services

DOI: 10.1057/9781137515445.0005

to this population as a whole—may make the mistake of thinking that by selecting against deafness, society is not only saying something negative about living with deafness but also something negative about deaf people. Given the available data on the socioeconomic impact of deafness, though, it is reasonable to infer that it is usually better to live without deafness than with deafness, but it is also reasonable for Deaf Pride advocates to assert that most hearing people have little understanding of deaf life and culture and thus are not in a position to make claims about what lives are better or worse. Here again, the process of counseling that is provided prior to the use of PGD can make an important contribution to well-informed and reasonable decision making on this difficult topic.

Another way in which selecting against deafness could negatively affect existing deaf people is through the shrinking effect it will have on the size of the deaf population, especially if PGD became more affordable and widespread in its use. In addition to there being a smaller community and potentially a decline in deaf culture, it may also be more difficult for a smaller deaf population to obtain educational or other important services.[25] Oftentimes, a critical mass of people is necessary for it to be profitable for an industry to provide certain goods and services. Therefore, the everyday lives of deaf people might actually be impacted by selection against deafness via PGD. However, if society prioritizes care for the deaf, for instance by subsidizing the manufacture of certain products for deaf people as part of the provision of Social Security disability benefits, it will still be possible to provide good quality care for a smaller deaf population. Thus if we deem deafness a sufficiently serious condition to warrant negative selection using PGD, we should not refrain from using PGD out of concern that people living with deafness will have decreased access to care.

Ultimately, the expressivist argument carries weight because we cannot entirely separate people's identities from their disabilities, particularly if their disability profoundly affects the communities to which they belong and other aspects of their culture, such as the language that they speak. However, concerns about the implications of selecting against a disability for existing disabled people cannot definitively outweigh parents' motivation to use PGD for this purpose—the desire to have a child without what may be considered a serious impairment. Thus the expressivist argument alone is not sufficient to justify prohibiting the use of PGD to select against deafness.

DOI: 10.1057/9781137515445.0005

Selecting for deafness

If we should not restrict parental choice to use PGD to select against deafness, how should we approach cases in which parents desire to select *for* deafness? Those who consider deafness to be a neutral variation may be comfortable with parents selecting for deaf children if our public policy protects a parental reproductive right to select for certain characteristics in their children. On the other hand, even if deafness is viewed as a value-neutral difference, we may object to this kind of nonmedical selection on other grounds.

One such ground for a policy that would not permit PGD to be used to select for deafness (or any disability) is the open future argument, which indeed was formulated specifically as an objection to selecting for deafness. Recall that Davis argues that selecting for deafness will reduce a future child's options, a claim that is supported by research on the relative socioeconomic status of deaf people and their families. The open future argument for reproductive decision making is perhaps only applicable in cases where parents desire to select for a disability, since it was not intended to be used to encourage parents to actively select against certain conditions or to encourage the use of PGD for enhancement purposes. As we previously noted, additional principles or moral considerations, such as those regarding humility, appropriate parenting, autonomy of the future person, and equitable access to expensive technology, must be used in conjunction with the open future argument so that in arguing against deliberating producing a deaf child with PGD it does not prove too much. The open future argument can also be used to support selection for other enhancing conditions, which, ironically, that may be precisely how some advocates view selection for deafness.

A powerful argument against using PGD to select for deafness is that doing so seriously harms the future child (if one believes that deafness is harmful to the affected person). One difficulty with this line of argument that we have not yet considered involves a philosophical puzzle about the relationship between harm and existence. This argument suggests that it is nearly impossible to harm a child by bringing it into existence because unless its life is so terrible that its suffering outweighs the benefit of existence, the child cannot be said to be worse off for having been born. By this reasoning, deliberately bringing a deaf child into the world is not harming the child because the deaf child is surely better off existing. If we compare the resulting child's life to some standard of normalcy

DOI: 10.1057/9781137515445.0005

or to some high standard of quality of life, then it may seem like a harm in the sense that it has forgone other possible traits and abilities. But if we compare the child's life to the alternative of never having a chance at life at all, the moral evaluation is different. This latter perspective is the nonidentity problem, and it permits a very wide spectrum of types of conditions that ethically prospective parents should be able to select for using PGD. For example, the nonidentity problem implies that a parent should be able to select for cystic fibrosis, because the parent is not harming the child unless we believe that people with cystic fibrosis would have been better off not living at all.

The same might be said of Huntington's disease. No one would use PGD to deliberately select for CF or Huntington's, though of course becoming pregnant itself poses a risk of having an affected child. How should we adjudicate between the opposite comparative perspectives of life versus nonexistence or limited life versus more highly enabled life? Some persons who know they are at risk for passing down the gene for Huntington's disease, for example, choose not to have children; others do so and take the 50–50 chance of having an affected child who will experience very difficult disabilities and have a foreshortened life span. At least until access to PGD is greatly increased, society must tolerate that cruel lottery. As serious as Huntington's is, we do not feel that living with it is worse than not existing at all.

While the nonidentity problem is baffling, we should not feel bound by its implications for two reasons. First, we can rely on other arguments unrelated to bringing harm to future children to justify limiting the use of PGD to select for disabilities or diseases (the arguments described previously relating to humility, autonomy, equal access, and the right to an open future). Second, focusing on whether or not selecting for a disability or disease can technically be considered harming a future child misses the point; we know that we should not deliberately create children who will be at a disadvantage or who will experience pain or suffering as a result of the selected condition, and that to do so would be to cause some kind of harm. Harm is usually applied to the case of doing something deleterious to an existing person; this is sometimes called "person-affecting" harm. But selecting for a disabling trait in an embryo will affect the person who is born and the subsequent life he or she leads, even if it is not a harm of this typical kind. In *From Chance to Choice*, Buchanan *et al.* suggest that selecting for a disabling condition involves harming in a different sense; it is a "non-person-affecting" harm, which does not do harm to a particular person so much as limit the range of choices in the life being created through the use of PGD-based selection for a disability.[26] In addition to appealing to a non-person-affecting, choice-limiting harm, we could also appeal to the distinction between a "harm" and a "wrong" and argue that selecting for a harmful condition is committing a wrongdoing, if not a direct harm.[27] In practice, then, it does not matter if our intuitions align with the metaphysical qualm raised by the nonidentity problem. Our intuitions are sufficiently clear and noncontroversial regarding conditions such as cystic fibrosis. As for deafness, the disagreement seems to lie in whether a deaf child is really disadvantaged or worse off, not in whether selecting a child who will be worse off is morally acceptable.

The question of allowing PGD to select for deafness thus hinges on whether a deaf child is worse off and whether we should allow nonmedical sex selection at all. Though it is conceivable that a deaf child who is afforded many social and educational opportunities would not experience deafness as a disadvantage, not every deaf child will have these advantages and the negative socioeconomic impact of deafness on the average deaf person has been demonstrated. Thus we are inclined to believe that deaf people are, on average, worse off in certain respects than those who can hear, and therefore that public policy should restrict the use of PGD to select for deaf children. On the grounds of the traditional rule of medical ethics, *primum non nocere* ("first, do no harm," or "above all, do not make matters worse"), it could also be argued that if we accept that deaf people are worse off, it would be unethical to use PGD for this purpose. And it would be a misuse of the medical art, whether or not a future deaf child could be said to have been harmed, because it is using medicine not to heal or to relieve suffering, but in the service of nonmedical values.

Adult onset diseases

Selection against adult onset diseases raises the question of what is a life worth living in a particularly acute manner. Is a life worth living if the first half can be normal and happy, until a latent disease begins to show symptoms? People with Huntington's disease, for example, can go to college, launch careers, start families, and have a major impact on those around them before the disease sets in, causing premature death

DOI: 10.1057/9781137515445.0005

at around 50 or 60 years of age. According to the expressivist argument, selection against Huntington's would send a negative message about people living with that condition. Others argue that "PGD may foster inaccurate identification of genes with disease and thus inadvertently reinforce problematic views of genetic causation and responsibility."[28] This is a reasonable concern, given common misconceptions regarding genetic determinism. Still others object to using PGD for adult onset diseases because some diseases have variable expressivity and penetrance and so genetic diagnosis will not tell us how severely a given individual will be affected later in life, or indeed, if a person will be symptomatic at all. Furthermore, we cannot predict whether treatment options will be available in the future, when a person with a late onset condition becomes affected by the disease.[29]

These concerns must be weighed against the desire to avoid passing on serious and deadly diseases that can cause great physical and emotional suffering later in life. Furthermore, we cannot take it for granted that people will live normal and happy lives until the symptoms of an adult onset disease begin to present themselves; it can be extremely stressful to live with the knowledge, or the foreboding and uncertainty, of having such a condition. On balance, the suffering caused by serious late onset diseases such as Huntington's or early onset Alzheimer's seem to place them squarely in the category of serious or severe diseases against which public policy ought to allow us to select via PGD.[30]

However, selection against diseases that only present themselves in the final years of life, such as late onset Alzheimer's (if something like PGD were ever to be able to identify a clear, actionable, genetic factor), may be less easily justified, since with such conditions the length of healthy life is much longer than the final decade or so in which disability is severe. Even then, subjective quality of life may not be terribly poor. Consider the balance of years without disease to years with disease in the case of a condition which is the reverse of Alzheimer's, such as ALS. With proper care and support, the quality and productivity of life with ALS can outweigh the suffering caused by the symptoms of the disease even in the final years or months of life. Parkinson's disease is yet another case in which these considerations are pertinent. Nonetheless, an argument can still be made that late onset Alzheimer's, ALS, and Parkinson's should certainly be prevented if possible, if not for the sake of the affected individual, then for the sake of family and other caregivers, and ultimately for society as a whole. Unfortunately, genetic science does not permit

DOI: 10.1057/9781137515445.0005

us to understand and predict these late onset conditions in the way we understand some of the early onset genetic conditions such as Tay Sachs or Lesch–Nyhan syndrome. The genetic factors of prevalent late onset conditions are too variable and the interaction between genomics and environmental factors is too complex. (This makes evolutionary sense because they are compatible with survival through at least the reproductive years.) But if we could predict Alzheimer's or ALS with PGD in the same way we can with early onset genetic disorders in children, then there would be a strong policy case for allowing for selection against such diseases in a preimplantation setting.

In many ways, "What is a life worth living?" is a risky question to ask because it emphasizes what the expressivist argument fears—that selecting against a particular condition is a comment on the worth of a life with that condition. Nevertheless, we cannot avoid this issue because using PGD *is* making a claim about what kinds of lives society views as better or worse. It is not that the moral worth of a diseased person is reduced; it is that living with a certain condition is worse than living without it, if all else is held equal. That remains true even if having the condition is not worse than not living at all. In this sense, PGD is more than a tool to facilitate private rights and choices. Our policy toward its use is a public commitment, a public endorsement of the technology. As such, PGD has different and sometimes conflicting implications for different groups of people. The governance of a public technology requires that we balance the interests of the future child, the family, specific populations, and society at large.

Savior siblings: creating one life for the sake of another

There are three main considerations weighing against using PGD to create savior siblings, or children who will serve as tissue donors for sick siblings. The first is that creating one life for the sake of another may constitute a violation of human dignity, since that child is being used as a means to the end of curing another child. The second is that the dependence of a child on his or her sibling as a tissue source may create strained family relations. The final consideration, mentioned in the introduction, is that PGD has not been available for long enough to properly assess the risks of embryo biopsy on the resulting child.[31] Thus when the sick

DOI: 10.1057/9781137515445.0005

sibling does not have a heritable disease that may also be present in the younger child and PGD is only performed for the sake of the older sibling, the younger child will bear the burden of the risks of embryo biopsy on behalf of his or her sibling.

The first consideration can be mitigated by the recognition that while the second child is being used as a means to an end, he or she is not being treated as a *mere* means. The humanity formulation of Kant's categorical imperative states that respect for persons requires that we never treat our humanity, or the aspect of humanity manifest in the individual person, as a means only. However, that principle does not preclude the possibility that persons are simultaneously means to the achievement of other ends and exemplars of humanity, with intrinsic value, who should be respected for their own sake, as ends in themselves.[32] Thus, it is possible to respect the humanity or dignity of savior siblings by valuing them in their own right, in addition to valuing them as tissue donors for their siblings.[33] This will likely be the case in most situations—the parents will be happy to have two healthy children rather than one sick child. However, it might be reasonable for parents to meet with a counselor or undergo a psychological screening process to examine their attitudes toward the future savior sibling.[34] Furthermore, younger siblings should not be used for tissues other than umbilical cord blood and bone marrow, the first of which is often discarded anyhow and the second of which is renewable.[35] Restricting the tissues that can be donated limits the *use* of the younger sibling, or the amount that he or she is treated as a means.

Precautionary measures could also be taken in order to address the second concern, that strained family relations will result from the dependence of the sick sibling on the savior sibling and the pressure on the savior sibling to donate tissue. For example, the number of times the donor sibling may be tested and materials may be harvested can be limited and psychological evaluations of the involved parties could take place before each new harvesting.[36]

Due to the nature of the procedure, we cannot alleviate the burden of the embryo biopsy's unknown risks to the savior sibling. However, we can ensure that the condition from which the sick sibling is suffering is severely debilitating or life-threatening in order to warrant PGD for HLA typing. This would stack the deck, so to speak, on the side of creating a savior sibling despite the relatively small risk that the embryo biopsy will harm the donor sibling.[37] The fact that one child will bear the

DOI: 10.1057/9781137515445.0005

risk burden for the other child is problematic, but if the risk to the donor sibling is sufficiently small, which is generally thought to be the case,[38] the risk may be outweighed by the ability to use donor tissue to heal a seriously ill person who is closely related to the donor sibling. Parents can and most likely will value donor children in their own right and treat them with the love and respect that they are due.

Elective sex selection

Sex selection is the primary way in which parents can and do select for nonmedical traits in their children, given the current capacities of PGD. Thus, the arguments described earlier against parents' choosing their children's characteristics are perhaps most applicable to elective sex selection in the near term. Yet sex selection also raises concerns that are separate from its classification as a nonmedical use of PGD, concerns regarding sex discrimination and stereotyping on both familial and societal levels.

Elective sex selection is frequently divided into two categories: (1) selection because parents simply prefer to have a child of one sex over the other, or (2) selection for the purpose of family balancing (having a child of the opposite sex as previous children). Whether there is a significant moral or practical difference between sex selection for family balancing or pure parental preference has been cast in doubt, however.[39] According to Stephen Wilkinson, the author of *Choosing Tomorrow's Children: The Ethics of Selective Reproduction*, people believe that sex selection is sexist because it reinforces either sex supremacy or sex stereotyping. It seems that both sex supremacy and stereotyping could play a role in selection for family balancing as well as in "regular" sex selection.[40] For example, parents with a supremacist preference for males over females could experience the misfortune of having several female children and desire to perform sex selection in order to have the male child they always desired. Regarding stereotyping, it seems likely that parents who strongly desire a child of a particular sex, even in addition to one of the opposite sex, hold opinions about the types of personalities that members of each sex will have and what it will be like to raise a child of each sex. This type of stereotyping can be considered sexist because it assumes that male and female children will have different personality types (e.g. aggressive and athletic vs. caring and musical[41]) and fill different roles from birth. Though sexist attitudes will not necessarily be present in parents who desire to use PGD for family balancing, they may likewise not be present in parents who want to carry out "regular" sex selection. It is not clear, then, why family balancing would be more justifiable than parental preference sex selection on the familial level.

Some argue that even though it is not necessarily less sexist, family balancing is preferable to parental preference sex selection because it has a more limited impact on population demographics. The worry is that sex selection via PGD could be used to reinforce a preference for male children, leading to a demographic imbalance like that in China and creating society-wide problems including increased rates of sexual violence and other crimes.[42] For those who believe that reproductive autonomy should not be restricted unless society at large may be harmed, it is important to distinguish between the familial and societal effects of a particular policy. If the problematic effects of family balancing are limited to the family, family balancing might be acceptable even if other forms of sex selection are not. However, it is not obvious that, even if family balancing has a relatively limited impact on population demographics, it would not have a negative impact nonetheless. If the population contains a roughly 50–50 male to female ratio and there were a societal preference for males, family balancing would be used to add more males to the population than females, thus throwing the male to female ratio out of balance.[43] While fewer people might gain access to sex selection if there were a family balancing rule, family balancing could still have a negative effect on demographics.

The primary consideration weighing in favor of allowing family balancing is that people have a right to reproductive autonomy and should be able to have a male or female child if they so choose. The reproductive rights argument could be made for other kinds of nonmedical sex selection as well, including selecting for a disability—why shouldn't a deaf couple be allowed to select for a deaf child if they want to? In the next chapter, we will examine arguments in favor of reproductive autonomy and its limitation in certain circumstances.

In the previous two chapters, we have attempted to present the major arguments for and against various uses of PGD, including the controversial applications mentioned in the introduction. We aimed to analyze the ethical issues in light of what is medically feasible and to determine which considerations are sufficiently well-grounded to weigh on the side of instituting regulations to limit certain uses of PGD. The following

DOI: 10.1057/9781137515445.0005

chapter will examine practical barriers to drafting and implementing PGD policy.

Notes

1   "Obesity Is Now a Disease, American Medical Association Decides." *Medical News Today*. MediLexicon International, August 17, 2013. Web. February 26, 2014.

2   Fryhofer, Sandra. *Is Obesity a Disease*. Rep. Vol. 3-A-13. American Medical Association, 2013. Report of the Council on Science and Public Health.

3   Ibid.

4   Ibid.

5   Ibid.

6   "Preimplantation Genetic Testing: A Practice Committee Opinion." *Fertility and Sterility* 90.5 (2008): S136–143.

7   *Reproduction and Responsibility: The Regulation of New Biotechnologies: A Report of the President's Council on Bioethics*. Washington, DC: President's Council on Bioethics, 2004.

8   *Beyond Therapy: Biotechnology and the Pursuit of Happiness: A Report of the President's Council on Bioethics*. Washington, DC: President's Council on Bioethics, 2003.

9   *Reproduction and Responsibility*. President's Council on Bioethics, 2004.

10   Two other factors to consider are how likely it is that a disease will present itself if a person has the associated gene and how likely it is that the symptoms will be severe. These are the concepts of penetrance and variable expressivity, respectively. Is it ethical to select against a condition if there is a 1% chance that a disease will result or that the resulting disease will be severe? What about 5%? Or 10%? The guidelines cited earlier do not provide definitive guidance on these issues, but it is logical that the justification for performing PGD would grow stronger as the risk that a disease will develop, and in a severe form, increases.

11   Scott, Rosamund. *Choosing between Possible Lives*. Oxford: Hart, 2007. Page 215.

12   Robertson, John. (2008) "Assisting Reproduction, Choosing Genes and the Scope of Reproductive Autonomy"; Pers. comm. Dr Mark Hughes, Founder and Director of Genesis Genetics, January 15, 2014.

13   Scott, Rosamund. *Choosing between Possible Lives*. Oxford: Hart, 2007. Page 26.

14   Pers. comm. Prof. Laura Mauldin, University of Connecticut, February 10, 2014; Marsha Saxton. "Why Members of the Disability Community Oppose Prenatal Diagnosis and Selective Abortion," in *Prenatal Testing and Disability*

DOI: 10.1057/9781137515445.0005

Rights. Erik Parens and Adrienne Asch, eds. Washington, DC: Georgetown UP, 2000. Pages 147–164.

15   Ibid. As an advocate for the reproductive rights of women, however, she is conflicted regarding whether or not PGD should be regulated to begin with.

16   Americans With Disabilities Act of 1990. Pub. L. 101–336. July 26, 1990. 104 Stat. 328.

17   Davis, Dena. (1997) "Genetic Dilemmas and the Child's Right to an Open Future."

18   Boss, Emily F., John K. Niparko, Darrell J. Gaskin, and Kimberly L. Levinson. "Socioeconomic Disparities for Hearing-Impaired Children in the United States." *The Laryngoscope* 121.4 (2011): 860–866.

19   Levi, N. "Deafness, Culture and Choice." *Journal of Medical Ethics* 28.5 (2002): 284–285.

20   Pers. comm. Prof. Leslie Francis, University of Utah, February 14, 2014.

21   Wilkinson, Stephen. *Choosing Tomorrow's Children: The Ethics of Selective Reproduction.* Oxford, England: Clarendon, 2010. Page 170.

22   Savulescu, Julian. (2001) "Procreative Beneficence: Why We Should Select the Best Children."

23   Murray, Thomas H. *The Worth of a Child.* Berkeley: University of California Press, 1996. Pages 131–132.

24   Given the difficulty of entirely separating people's identities from their disabilities, Savulescu's claim that we should select against disabilities because it will result in better off people is problematic for him as a utilitarian, as maximizing the overall well-being requires that utilitarians value the lives of the better off more than the lives of the worse off. In other words, Savulescu actually *would* value the lives of deaf people less than those of hearing people, though he would not advocate that we treat the deaf with less respect.

25   Pers. comm. Prof. Leslie Francis, University of Utah, February 14, 2014.

26   Buchanan, Allen E., Dan W. Brock, Norman Daniels, and Daniel Wikler. *From Chance to Choice: Genetics and Justice.* Cambridge, UK: Cambridge UP, 2000. Pages 247–255.

27   Ibid. Pages 234; 250–253.

28   Ethics Committee of the American Society for Reproductive Medicine. "Use of Preimplantation Genetic Diagnosis for Serious Adult Onset Conditions: A Committee Opinion." *Fertility and Sterility* 100 (2013): 54–57.

29   Baruch, S. (2009) "Preimplantation Genetic Diagnosis and Parental Preferences: Beyond Deadly Disease."

30   Ethics Committee of the American Society for Reproductive Medicine. (2013) "Use of Preimplantation Genetic Diagnosis for Serious Adult Onset Conditions: A Committee Opinion."

31   Ibid.

DOI: 10.1057/9781137515445.0005

32   Kant, Immanuel. *The Moral Law, or, Kant's Groundwork of the Metaphysic of Morals: A New Translation with Analysis and Notes.* Trans. H. J. Paton. New York: Barnes & Noble, 1956. Page 96.

33   Wolf, Susan, Jeffrey Kahn, and John Wagner. "Using Preimplantation Genetic Diagnosis to Create a Stem Cell Donor: Issues, Guidelines & Limits." *Journal of Law, Medicine and Ethics* 31 (2003): 327–339.

34   Ibid.

35   *Preimplantation Tissue Typing: Policy Review.* Rep.: Human Fertilisation and Embryology Authority, 2004.

36   Wolf *et al.* (2003) "Using Preimplantation Genetic Diagnosis to Create a Stem Cell Donor: Issues, Guidelines & Limits."

37   Ibid.

38   Ethics Committee of the American Society for Reproductive Medicine. (2013) "Use of Preimplantation Genetic Diagnosis for Serious Adult Onset Conditions: A Committee Opinion."

39   Wilkinson, Stephen. *Choosing Tomorrow's Children: The Ethics of Selective Reproduction.* Page 222.

40   Ibid. Pages 223–226.

41   Ibid. Page 226.

42   Edlund, Lena, Hongbin Li, Junjian Yi, and Junsen Zhang. "Sex Ratios and Crime: Evidence from China." *The Review of Economics and Statistics* 95.5 (2013): 1520–1534.

43   Wilkinson, Stephen. *Choosing Tomorrow's Children: The Ethics of Selective Reproduction.* Page 221.

DOI: 10.1057/9781137515445.0005

4

Regulating PGD in Practice

Abstract: *In this chapter, we discuss the two major sociolegal concepts relating to the regulation of PGD in practice: the importance of reproductive autonomy and the fear that embryo selection will return us to an era of eugenics. We then present the various levels at which PGD might be regulated, culminating in a summary of the pros and cons of government regulation vs. professional self-regulation. The UK's Human Fertilisation and Embryology Authority's system for regulating PGD is offered as one example of how policy can be developed in this scientific and moral gray area. The chapter concludes with a presentation of available data on both public and professional opinion regarding the appropriate uses and limitations of PGD. The "bottom line" is that in order to answer the question "should PGD be more regulated?", we must first decide whether the present state of self-regulation is sufficient, which in turn depends on our views regarding government involvement in medical practice, reproductive autonomy, and whether or not current uses of PGD are morally troubling.*

Bayefsky, Michelle and Bruce Jennings. *Regulating Preimplantation Genetic Diagnosis in the United States: The Limits of Unlimited Selection.* New York: Palgrave Macmillan, 2015. DOI: 10.1057/9781137515445.0006.

The ethical issues raised in Chapters 2 and 3 comprise many of the important considerations regarding whether or not PGD ought to be regulated in the United States, but they must be weighed against legal and social obstacles to generating PGD policy. In this chapter, we will introduce and discuss the major considerations that remain: procreative autonomy and the legitimacy of government intervention, concerns related to the history of eugenics in the United States, and the pros and cons of the various regulatory options. We do not aim to provide a conclusive justification for PGD regulation or a detailed blueprint for the form that a regime of PGD governance and regulation should take. Instead, we shall try to advance the ongoing policy discussion by reviewing the views of different stakeholders, including physicians, genetic counselors, bioethicists, and members of the public, and by examining various policy and action implications of their beliefs and interests.

Reproductive autonomy and its limits

Regulation in the area of reproduction has been controversial in the United States because of its proximity to the abortion debate and because of the history of eugenics, both of which raise important questions about procreative freedom. Just as it is important to examine the ethical implications of allowing certain uses of PGD, it is crucial that PGD regulations not unjustly impinge on people's right to reproductive autonomy. In the past, reproductive rights debates have centered on the freedom to reproduce or not reproduce.[1] The availability of assisted reproductive technologies that allow us to choose certain characteristics in children introduces the question of *what kind* of children we should be able to have, and how much control we should have in the matter. Despite this shift in focus, it is nevertheless useful to review previous cases related to reproductive rights in order to see how US law has approached the concept of reproductive autonomy and its limitation.

Two major cases that relate to the right to have children are the *Buck vs. Bell* and *Skinner v. Oklahoma* cases. In the 1927 *Buck* case, the US Supreme Court sanctioned the compulsory sterilization of "mental defectives."[2] Chief Justice Holmes wrote in the decision that sterilization would promote both the patient's welfare and that of society; the combination justified the limitation of the reproductive rights of those deemed to be "imbeciles."[3] While the decision was never overturned, it

DOI: 10.1057/9781137515445.0006

is widely viewed as reflective of the eugenicist ideas that were pervasive at the time and have since been disavowed.[4] By contrast, in the 1942 *Skinner* case, the Supreme Court held that forced sterilization could not be used as punishment for recidivist criminals. The decision mentioned a "basic...right to have offspring" but primarily relied on the specifics of Oklahoma's law, which was said to violate the Equal Protection Clause.[5] Nevertheless, *Skinner* was an important step toward establishing a right to be able to have children.

The 1965 Supreme Court case *Griswold v. Connecticut* is often cited as a landmark case in the establishment of reproductive rights. In *Griswold*, the Court struck down Connecticut's contraceptive ban on the grounds that the law violated a "right to marital privacy."[6] Though it only applied to married couples, the decision was significant in that it linked reproductive rights to the concept of privacy and asserted that married couples should be able to have children, or not have children, as they saw fit.

Roe v. Wade built on the concept of privacy in reproductive matters, this time regarding individual women. The decision established a constitutional right to an abortion in at least the first trimester of pregnancy based on a woman's right to "personal privacy."[7] Justice Blackmun noted in the decision, however, that the right to privacy should not be viewed as absolute. He wrote that the state "may properly assert important interests in safeguarding health, in maintaining medical standards, and in protecting potential life." At "some point in pregnancy, these respective interests become sufficiently compelling to sustain regulation of the factors that govern the abortion decision."[8] Thus, the state may limit the right to terminate a pregnancy if it can demonstrate that it has a sufficiently compelling interest in doing so.

The major cases cited earlier illustrate that in US case law, there is an accepted right to reproductive autonomy, generally based on a right to privacy, but that this right is not absolute. As Robertson writes, "most liberties are presumptive rights," meaning that they "are protected unless there are sufficiently weighty interests on the other side."[9] It is also unclear how the right to decide whether and when to have children would translate into questions about what kinds of children we should be able to have. Robertson concludes that while the "freedom to screen, identify, and perhaps even alter genes should follow from the standard accounts of reproductive autonomy," the scope of this freedom has yet to be determined. The right to personal privacy seems relevant to the

DOI: 10.1057/9781137515445.0006

freedom to choose children's characteristics, but how far does it extend and what state interests could justify its limitation?

Robertson asserts that reproductive choices regarding children's characteristics "must be plausibly related to societal understandings of reproduction and why it is important, not simply a desire to use reproductive components in particular ways."[10] Why reproduction is important is a broad category, though, and may include a wide range of personal and cultural beliefs that would need to be vetted and approved. Perhaps we could rule out selection for superficial traits such as eye and hair color using Robertson's standard, but those applications are not likely to be available in the near future, if at all. Extremely trivial or idiosyncratic reasons to utilize PGD will always be disproportional to the financial cost and medical risk or inconvenience. Meanwhile, selection for deafness, sex, and many other less "superficial" traits could relatively easily be construed to fit within his conception of reproductive autonomy.

Many of the arguments explored in the previous chapters could be used to justify a compelling state interest in restricting the use of PGD, at least for some purposes. With regard to selection for deafness, if the state can assert an interest in protecting future life, it may be able to assert an interest in protecting the quality of that future life.[11] Therefore, if we decide that deafness leads to a lower quality of life for the average deaf person, at least in certain respects, the state might regulate PGD selection for deafness (or other arguably disabling conditions) on this basis. It would also be useful to apply the category of "harm" to selecting for a disability when establishing a compelling state interest, but as we have seen, in the PGD domain the nonidentity problem makes applying a straightforward conception of harm more complicated than it ordinarily is in legal, ethical, or policy analysis. To circumvent this issue, we could employ the broader category of wrongdoing or we could argue that a harm is being caused and the future child experiences it, even if the future child is not being harmed directly unless a particular condition is generally viewed as worse than death. Aside from harm or wrongdoing, the state could also claim an interest in protecting the autonomy of future children. Joel Feinberg and Dena Davis argued for a *legal* right to an open future, and advocated for restrictions on the decisions that parents could make on behalf of their children before they reach maturity. The legal right to an open future could thus be used to justify a compelling state interest in limiting the use of PGD to select for disabilities.

DOI: 10.1057/9781137515445.0006

A state interest in protecting the autonomy of the future child could also be used to restrict nonmedical uses of PGD more generally, including sex selection. While the number of options available to the future child would not necessarily be fewer when parents select for non-disease-related traits, we argued in Chapter 2 that autonomy for children also requires that parents not overly determine their genetic characteristics.

Rather than claiming an interest in the rights of future children, other arguments supporting a state interest in limiting certain uses of PGD relate to their impact on society at large. For example, the possibility of creating a demographic shift toward one sex or the other, and all the associated problems, could be used to restrict elective sex selection,[12] even for family balancing. In the short term, however, given the physical and financial burden of performing IVF and PGD, it is extremely unlikely that enough people would carry out elective sex selection via PGD to cause a demographic shift. Evidence also suggests that overall PGD use in the United States does not favor one sex over the other.[13] However, as noted earlier, it has been reported that within certain Asian and Middle Eastern subpopulations in the United States, elective sex selection has been utilized to select predominantly for males.[14] Sex selection against female embryos can be viewed as both a sexist action in itself, as well as a reinforcement of sexist attitudes and discriminatory behaviors toward existing women.[15] Thus, a state interest could be established on the grounds that elective sex selection constitutes and reinforces sexism and sex discrimination.

Society-level arguments for restricting the use of PGD can also be made in financial terms. Specifically, providing services to children and adults with disabilities is financially burdensome on society, since some care will be funded by the Social Security system. Thus selecting for a disability not only affects the future child and the community of people with that disability, but also generates an additional cost for everyone in society. It is unlikely that policy arguments against selecting for deaf children would be framed in these terms, however, given the discomfort many people feel with assigning monetary values to different kinds of lives.

Another ethical value and state interest that pertains to the governance of PGD is justice and equity of access to the technology. Moreover, social equality more broadly, not merely equity of access, is at stake. For example, if we were to reach the point at which advantages such as strength and intelligence could be selected via PGD, allowing such uses

DOI: 10.1057/9781137515445.0006

could exacerbate inequalities and even create different strata of people based on their genes (like in the movie Gattaca).[16] It is also paradoxical, to say the least, to contemplate allocating resources for inequitable enhancement uses of PGD, when a basic, universal system to prevent disease using PGD does not exist. However, this enhancement scenario is very unlikely given the limitations of genetic and reproductive medical technology. Furthermore, as will be discussed in the next chapter, in the highly voluntaristic and market-oriented governance regime for PGD now in place in the United States, inequitable access to PGD already exists given the high price of fertility treatment and general lack of insurance coverage for IVF.

Other arguments raised in the previous chapter, though legitimate, would be difficult to translate into compelling state interests that would justify restricting access to certain uses of PGD. For example, concerns regarding the importance of humility toward nature and the potential for nonmedical sex selection to encourage problematic approaches to parenting are based on particular notions of what constitutes a good attitude toward life and parenting. For the state to limit the use of PGD on the basis of these concerns would be to impose a particular worldview regarding very personal and subjective matters. Furthermore, the expressivist argument regarding the message that negative selection might send to people with disabilities, while reasonable, is not sufficient to justify banning the use of PGD to select against certain disabilities. Instead, we should take appropriate measures to ensure that people with disabilities are properly respected and receive the care that they need.

A final society-level concern that might favor governmental regulation of PGD is an interest in the well-being of the shared gene pool. The DNA of every person belongs to a common pool from which future generations are formed. The gene pool concept helps to explain the intuition that therapies like PGD, which affect the germline, are fundamentally different from ones that affect only somatic cells.[17] Treatment decisions that impact the germline have an effect that can persist for generations into the future, generations that are common to everyone, and thus are often viewed as having a greater impact on society at large.[18] The government could articulate an interest in the well-being of the gene pool if it felt that the use of PGD was altering the gene pool in a way that threatened the good of society. However, as noted earlier regarding sex selection, PGD would have to be significantly more common in order for the state to assert a legitimate interest in the overall genetic makeup

DOI: 10.1057/9781137515445.0006

of the population. Furthermore, using the concept of the gene pool to justify the limitation of reproductive autonomy is problematic because it is reminiscent of eugenics-era notions of perfecting the human race for the sake of the common good. Thus while modifications of the shared gene pool can, in an abstract sense, be said to affect all of its members, it is unclear what kinds of restrictions of reproductive autonomy could reasonably stem from a state interest in protecting the gene pool.

Like reproductive freedom, the state interests described earlier are not absolute but must be weighed against other considerations. When determining whether to limit reproductive autonomy by restricting certain uses of PGD, regulators cannot simply say, "sex selection is sexist" or "non-medical PGD violates the autonomy of the future child." Instead, they must ask: What are the social effects of sexually biased practices in this particular domain and context? Should this level of sexism or bias be tolerated if it has little demonstrable impact on future children, specific subpopulations, and society as a whole?[19] What are the costs of restricting a discriminatory practice such as this and do those costs exceed the benefits of regulation or prohibition? Once these issues are fully explored, we might conclude that despite the problematic motivations and ramifications of some uses of elective sex selection, for example, the right to make reproductive decisions freely is more important. Furthermore, we must be wary of the historical and social implications of the arguments that we use to justify state intervention into reproductive matters.

Eugenics and its implications for PGD

What is "eugenics" and does the history of its practice pose an obstacle to the regulation of PGD? As Wilkinson notes, what is commonly meant by "eugenics" exists on a continuum between "authoritarian" eugenics and "laissez-faire" eugenics.[20] The former implies a certain level of coercion, as was characteristic of compulsory sterilization by the Nazis, while the latter indicates that parental choice in a free market dictates children's genes. However, in our view, such a broad definition of eugenics is not helpful and flies in the face of deeply engrained usage. The "laissez-faire" end of Wilkinson's spectrum, the private choices and preferences of parents, as long as they are not the result of wrongful pressure or coercion, is not best thought of as eugenics at all, precisely because they are private decisions, while eugenics is a public system of values and

DOI: 10.1057/9781137515445.0006

practices which expresses itself at a more general level of culture and society. We typically think of eugenics as "authoritarian," coercive, and bigoted, and the aspects of authority or power here are not simply one end of a continuum but are inherent in the practice as such in all of its various forms. Eugenics as a public expression of certain norms, and as an application of social power over defiance and difference, has made terrible mistakes. We now know that Carrie Buck, whose involuntary sterilization under the Virginia Sterilization Act (1924) was upheld by the Supreme Court in *Buck v. Bell*, was not developmentally disabled at all, but was the victim of abuse at the hands of the law and medicine.[21] There is little wonder then, that those who support the use of PGD, at least in certain circumstances, object to the comparison of PGD to eugenics. PGD, they say, has nothing to do with coercion and is an expression of reproductive choice rather than the subjugation of choice. Critics of PGD and other genetic manipulations may or may not believe that these procedures are carried out under coercive circumstances, but they recognize that using the term "eugenics" is an effective weapon because its authoritarian connotations cast a pall over the entire enterprise.[22]

Coercive eugenics, including forced sterilization or the breeding of humans, is now universally viewed as an immoral and unacceptable breach of personal autonomy and human rights. People object to both the coercive and brutal means by which authoritarian eugenics has been practiced and the ends of eugenics—to improve the "stock" of the human population.[23] Historically, eugenics was used to provide medical legitimacy to racism; there was no scientific basis for claims about what groups of people were "better" or "worse" and should therefore not be able to contribute their genes to the next generation. Thus three distinct problems with authoritarian eugenics can be identified and used to assess whether regulating PGD will be similarly problematic: (1) the means of coercion, (2) the society-level assessment of what constitutes a "better" or "worse" gene, and (3) the restriction of the reproductive autonomy of members of the population via the imposition of the values laid out in (2).[24]

Before applying these three problems to the use and regulation of PGD, it will be helpful to mention the distinction that is often made between positive and negative eugenics. Positive eugenics is typically viewed as selection for specific traits, or enhancement, whereas negative eugenics has been used to refer to selection against undesirable conditions, including disease. Many view this distinction to be morally significant and believe that positive eugenics is worse than negative eugenics.[25] It is

DOI: 10.1057/9781137515445.0006

unclear, however, whether a line can really be drawn between positive and negative selection. Selecting against Tay Sachs is selecting for a child without Tay Sachs, for instance. Furthermore, by the definition cited earlier, the use of PGD to select against severe diseases would be classified as negative eugenics. The distinction we have used between medical and nonmedical uses of PGD cuts across the positive eugenics and negative eugenics distinction, if by positive we mean an intention to enhance and by negative we mean an intention to prevent. Some medical uses may be enhancing rather than simply preventative. Some nonmedical uses may be described as preventative. In using these terms, the significance and moral evaluation hinges on the nature of the alternative being forgone and the character of the baseline against which the goals of genetic selection are being measured. It is the difference between trying to prevent an individual from falling far below the species typical norm of functioning and trying to provide the genetic basis for an individual to far exceed the typical level of functioning. Eugenics for either preventative or enhancement purposes—no more "idiots" or outstanding athletes—and whether pursued by medical or nonmedical means—sterilization or genetically guided marriage—is ethically suspect today.[26]

The three issues mentioned are useful precisely because of this difficulty in determining what constitutes eugenics; it doesn't matter what you call it if you find it problematic by one or more of the three criteria. Different kinds of PGD policies may be considered problematic depending on their nature and how they are applied. For example, to require that a couple with dwarfism who is already undergoing IVF and PGD select only those embryos that will result in a child of normal stature would be an inappropriate means of coercion.[27] Another coercive use of state power might involve providing fiscal or social incentives to selecting for a child without a certain disease or disability. These cases are problematic because they use PGD policy to pressure or compel people to carry out PGD, rather than describe when PGD may be performed if people so choose.

Regulations that delineate when PGD *may* be carried out, as distinct from those that dictate when it should be used, while not coercive, could nevertheless be criticized on the grounds that they assert a particular view of what genes are better or worse.[28] This is the expressivist argument discussed previously in the context of allowing parents to select against deafness. While the expressivist argument contains merit because it is difficult to separate some people's identities from their disabilities, it is much stronger when applied to regulations *requiring* particular uses of PGD

DOI: 10.1057/9781137515445.0006

rather than regulations that simply permit people to use PGD. It seems to be the combination of coercive tactics and normative claims about what constitutes a better or worse life, linked to notions of how different lives should be valued, that we find particularly objectionable about eugenics. Furthermore, the content of eugenicists' normative claims tended to be racist and unscientific—the value judgments they made were often based on inaccurate measures of quality of life anyhow. In order to avoid the charge of eugenics, PGD regulations must be firmly based on evidence about the impact of having certain genes on measures of quality of life.

The third criterion listed earlier regards reproductive autonomy. As mentioned in the previous section, eugenics was used to restrict reproductive choice by forbidding some people from procreating, which is different from forbidding people from choosing particular characteristics in their children. Nevertheless, we ought to take the limitation of reproductive freedom seriously, especially if we are considering very restrictive regulations that prohibit the use of PGD even for serious or severe conditions. In this case, banning PGD would amount to forbidding some people from having children altogether, if they would not have a child with such a condition.[29] An outright ban of PGD, or prohibiting the use of PGD for severe conditions, can thus be deemed problematic because of its restriction of the freedom to reproduce for carriers of severe disease.

Some kinds of PGD policies, in particular those that restrict reproduction completely for certain people and those that require certain uses of PGD, would be objectionable for some of the same reasons that we find eugenics objectionable. However, limiting the use of PGD in other ways (e.g. prohibiting sex selection or selection for a disability), while impinging on reproductive autonomy (as discussed in the previous section), cannot legitimately be called a eugenic use of state power. While it is important to be wary of the state exercising excessive control over what kind of children we can and cannot choose to have via the regulation of PGD, our concerns should generally center on reproductive autonomy and its limitations rather than comparisons of PGD regulation to eugenics.

Options for regulation

We turn now to an outline of several mechanisms by which PGD could be regulated along with potential obstacles to their successful

DOI: 10.1057/9781137515445.0006

implementation. In order to avoid the critiques presented earlier, none of these regulations would involve banning PGD outright or requiring that it be used in certain cases. Instead, they would limit the use of PGD for specific purposes or define when PGD is permitted. For example, they might prohibit sex selection or selection for a disability, or they might limit the use of PGD to selection against serious conditions.

There are a number of governing or regulatory bodies which may be relevant to the regulation of PGD: Congress, the Food and Drug Administration (FDA), the Centers for Disease Control and Prevention (CDC), the Centers for Medicare and Medicaid Services (CMS), state legislatures, and professional societies including the American Society for Reproductive Medicine (ASRM), the American College of Medical Genetics (ACMG), and the American Congress of Obstetricians and Gynecologists (ACOG). There are benefits and drawbacks to regulating PGD through all of these bodies, which will be discussed further on.

The US Congress could pass a law outlining acceptable and unacceptable uses of PGD. One advantage to passing such a law at the federal level is that there would be uniformity in access to particular uses of PGD across the country; someone could not select for sex in California but not in Texas, for example. However, Congress does not generally intervene in private medical practice by directly regulating the ways in which medical technologies are used.[30] Furthermore, it is extremely unlikely, particularly with the current divisive climate, that Congress would be able to pass legislation on such a sensitive ethical issue. Not only does PGD touch upon questions of what constitutes a disease or disability and whether reproductive freedom can be limited in the case of embryo selection, but it also lies perilously close to the contentious abortion debate.[31] PGD, like IVF, requires creating embryos, some of which will be discarded (if they are not frozen for later use or for donation). PGD also adds the additional complication that some embryos will be discarded because they carry an unwanted condition, which some find problematic.[32] In order for Congress to devise regulations for the use of PGD, it would have to assign responsibility for the embryos that would be discarded in the process of carrying out PGD, but to whom? The IVF program? Some newly created custodial agency? This approach would most likely be politically infeasible, since Congress would be unable to agree on the appropriate fate of excess embryos.

The FDA is responsible for ensuring the safety and efficacy of drugs and medical devices in the United States, including the drugs and

DOI: 10.1057/9781137515445.0006

devices employed in IVF and PGD. For example, the FDA approved of the hormones administered during fertility treatment and as mentioned in the introduction, has also approved of a new Illumina, Inc. gene sequencer that can be used to test for any gene. The FDA is also responsible for regulating the claims that companies make about its products, including genetic testing products. In November 2013, for instance, the FDA sent a letter to the genetic testing company 23andMe, Inc. demanding that they stop marketing their Personal Genome Service because it had not been granted marketing clearance for the claims that it was making regarding the health information the service could provide to consumers.[33] Although the FDA guarantees the safety and efficacy of medical drugs and devices, it does not have the authority to regulate how doctors use or administer medical products.[34,35] Thus it would be not be within the FDA's authority to approve gene sequencers or genetic tests with the caveat that they only be used for certain applications.

In addition to drugs and devices, the FDA regulates human issues intended for transplantation, including embryos that are created for transfer into a woman's uterus.[36] However, the FDA's oversight is limited to preventing the transmission of communicable disease, ensuring that tissues are properly tested and stored, and requiring that records be properly maintained.[37] While it may be tempting to suggest that the FDA define "communicable disease" in such a way that includes the transmission of serious hereditary disorders, the intention of the law is to prevent the transplant recipient—in this case, the prospective mother—from contracting communicable diseases such as chlamydia and gonorrhea.[38] Furthermore, it would be practically difficult for the FDA to regulate PGD through its control over tissue transplantation because it does not regulate fertility treatment protocols or the operation of fertility clinics.[39]

The CDC does not regulate the operation of fertility clinics either, but it is responsible for implementing the 1992 Fertility Clinic Success Rate and Certification Act (FCSRA), which requires that fertility clinics annually report pregnancy rates resulting from the various treatments that they offer (e.g. IVF, intracytoplasmic sperm injection (ICSI), fresh and frozen embryo transfers). The CDC publishes this information in an annual ART report, which is the primary source of data on the use of ART in the United States. While PGD usage has been included in the report in recent years, the reason why it was used has not been part of the collected data—only whether or not it was performed as part of an

DOI: 10.1057/9781137515445.0006

IVF cycle.[40] The CDC's relation to PGD is thus restricted to reporting its usage, and only in a limited sense.

CMS is involved in the use of PGD because it is responsible for developing and enforcing the Clinical Laboratory Improvement Amendments (CLIA), which regulate clinical laboratories. The CLIA rules ensure that testing, including genetic testing, is performed in accredited labs by qualified personnel who carry out approved protocols with calibrated instruments and appropriate reagents. CLIA also regulates specimen collection and processing, test orders and result reporting, and in such a way that does not compromise specimen integrity or patient confidentiality.[41] Like the FDA and CDC, however, CLIA does not regulate the practice of medicine, or what clinical laboratories can and cannot test for. Therefore, CMS is not in a good position to regulate the conditions for which PGD may be used.

The CLIA standards are also used in the accreditation process of the Joint Commission on Accreditation of Healthcare Organizations (JCAHO), which is one of the two primary ways in which fertility clinics are certified.[42] This means that the ability of the Joint Commission to regulate PGD through clinic certification is similarly limited to quality assurance. (The other major accrediting process is the College of American Pathologists/American Society for Reproductive Medicine (CAP/ASRM) accreditation program, which is aimed at "improving the quality of laboratory services through voluntary participation, professional peer review, education and compliance with established performance standards."[43] In other words, clinics can be certified via self-regulation, which will be discussed later.)

If the existing, relevant federal agencies are not well suited for the regulation of PGD, it would be possible to devise a new federal agency to deal specifically with the regulation of reproductive medical technology. Such an agency would be similar to the UK's HFEA, which is charged with the task of setting standards for and issuing licenses to UK fertility centers, as well as determining policies for fertility treatments including PGD.[44] This agency could generate and enforce clear regulations for the use of PGD. In theory, creating a new federal agency would also avoid the difficulty of passing controversial legislation. However, it is hard to imagine the current divided Congress, particularly one that has struggled with budgeting, agreeing on the creation and scope of such an agency. Perhaps most importantly, the US federal government generally does not involve itself in private medical practice to this degree.[45] As mentioned in

DOI: 10.1057/9781137515445.0006

the introduction, one reason the HFEA is responsible for regulating the conditions for which PGD may be used is that it must determine which uses of PGD the NHS should fund. In the United States, by contrast, the government is not the primary insurer of most American citizens and Medicare and Medicaid do not cover fertility treatment. Thus, it would be extremely unusual for a new federal agency to be created in order to regulate the practice of fertility specialists and ensure that PGD was only used for certain purposes.

State legislatures, by contrast, have traditionally held considerable authority over the practice of medicine.[46] Though no state has passed a law directly addressing PGD, some states have passed laws related to ART—on gestational surrogacy and gamete donation, for example. States can limit medical practice if they can demonstrate that doing so would benefit public health or safety; in other words, if they can show that they have a compelling state interest that justifies intervening in the doctor–patient relationship and restricting the reproductive autonomy of its citizens.[47] Regulating at the state level also seems more feasible than regulating at the federal level because it may be easier to achieve agreement on the appropriate uses of PGD at the state level. However, state-by-state regulation will result in variable PGD policy throughout the country. One state may allow elective sex selection, for instance, while another state bans the use of PGD for all but the most serious conditions. Bioethical issues often result in varied regulations around the country, though, and there are positives and negatives to the federalist approach.[48] However, there is no doubt that variable laws will create inconsistencies in people's ability to access PGD for different uses, inconsistencies that will be exacerbated by the fact that some people can afford to travel to another state for treatment while others cannot.

At the state level, there is also the troubling prospect that a legislature might pass a law that bans PGD outright. Even though such a Draconian measure would constitute a serious violation of the reproductive autonomy of couples who need to use PGD in order to have healthy children to whom they are genetically related, it could take years for such a ban to be struck down by a court. In the meantime, couples in that state, particularly couples without the means to travel to another state for care, will have been denied access to the fertility treatment that they require. This is an ethical risk of health governance in a federal system; states may be in the best position to regulate medical practice, but they may also be

DOI: 10.1057/9781137515445.0006

the most likely to legislate based on strong ideological views regarding the moral status of embryos and popular fears about designer babies.

The final option for regulating PGD is through self-regulation by professional societies. Professional organizations such as the ASRM, ACOG, and ACMG are well suited to regulating the practice of their members in the fertility, OB/GYN and genetics fields since they are best acquainted with patient needs and the day-to-day challenges of medical practice. However, unlike federal or state regulation, professional guidelines are not legally binding, though practitioners are more vulnerable to court action if they do not follow the standards of practice set by their professional societies. It is also important to keep in mind that professional organizations represent their members—medical practitioners and laboratory technicians in a particular subspecialty—first and foremost, and regulation generally makes their work more difficult (with regard to filling out paperwork and ensuring that they are complying with all the stipulations of a new policy).

Furthermore, the views of members of medical societies in the area of reproductive medicine may not always reflect the views of the American populace, particularly as they relate to matters of reproductive autonomy. For example, a 2009 ACOG Committee on Health Care for Underserved Women opinion calls abortion "an integral component of women's reproductive health services" and states that "the American College of Obstetricians and Gynecologists supports availability of reproductive health services for all women."[49] By contrast, a 2013 Gallup poll indicates that 58% of Americans believe abortion should be illegal in all (20%) or in all but a few (38%) circumstances.[50] Though there are no available polling data comparing the views of ASRM, ACOG, and ACMG members on the various uses of PGD to those of the general public, it would not be surprising if medical practitioners were more permissive than the public at large. Therefore, it is necessary to balance the valuable expertise and experience of physicians in this area with concerns about whether their moral views represent the American populace as a whole.[51]

The American Society for Reproductive Medicine has published several opinions relevant to the use of PGD. In 1999, the ASRM Ethics Committee recommended that PGD for elective sex selection be discouraged on the basis that it holds a "risk of unwarranted gender bias, social harm, and the diversion of medical resources from genuine medical need."[52] A 2001 Ethics Committee Opinion on the use of sperm sorting for sex selection recommended that it be used preliminarily for

DOI: 10.1057/9781137515445.0006

family balancing, and only subsequently for other nonmedical uses if the "social, psychological, and demographic effects" have been deemed acceptable.[53] The ASRM Ethics Committee met in September 2014 to reconsider its guidelines on sex selection and a new opinion will likely be published in the near future. According to Dr Paula Amato, the Chair of the ASRM Ethics Committee, the committee was unable to reach a consensus on whether or not elective sex selection should be considered ethically permissible and will recommend that individual doctors and clinics decide whether to offer this service.[54]

Two other relevant ASRM documents are a 2008 Practice Committee opinion on preimplantation genetic testing and a 2013 Ethics Committee opinion on the use of PGD for serious adult onset conditions. The Practice Committee document lists as indications for performing PGD "risk for transmitting a specific genetic disease or abnormality," carrying "mutations such as BRCA-1 that do not cause a specific disease but are thought to confer significantly increased risk for a disease" and "human leukocyte antigen (HLA) matching...in conjunction with testing for a specific genetic mutation."[55] Though PGD is recommended for these reasons, the ASRM guidelines do not limit PGD to these uses and no comments were included either encouraging or discouraging the use of PGD for other purposes. The 2013 Ethics Committee document is prefaced with the statement: "While this document reflects the views of members of that Committee, it is not intended to be the only approved standard of practice or to dictate an exclusive course of treatment in all cases." The opinion concludes that PGD for adult onset conditions is "ethically justifiable when the conditions are serious and when there are no known interventions for the conditions or the available interventions are either inadequately effective or significantly burdensome." Such a definition would include the use of PGD for the BRCA genes, for example, since prophylactic mastectomy is clearly a burdensome procedure. The opinion further specifies that "For conditions that are less serious or of lower penetrance, PGD for adult onset conditions is ethically acceptable as a matter of reproductive liberty," but emphasizes that the long-term effects of embryo biopsy are largely unknown.[56] Thus, medical practitioners should pause before, but ultimately allow, the use of PGD for less serious conditions.

In summary, the ASRM recommendations for the use of PGD do not prescribe when the technique should and should not be used, both because the opinions are not sufficiently specific and because they are not intended to dictate practice. Rather, published and unpublished committee documents suggest that medical practitioners should have some flexibility regarding the applications of PGD that they feel comfortable using and patients should be afforded leeway in the use of PGD in the name of reproductive liberty.

The American Congress of Obstetricians and Gynecologists has also published several policy statements that are relevant to the use of PGD. For example, in 2008, the Ethics and Genetics Committees published a joint opinion on ethical issues in genetic testing. Like the ASRM document cited earlier, the opinion is prefaced with the statement: "The information should not be construed as dictating an exclusive course of treatment or procedure to be followed." The document recommends that preconception and prenatal screening (not preimplantation screening) be used for a "limited number of severe child-onset diseases because such...testing provides individuals with the chance to pursue assisted reproductive technology in order to avoid conception of an affected child, to consider termination of a pregnancy, or to prepare for the birth of a chronically ill child." The statement also mentions new selective capabilities afforded specifically by the use of PGD, including selection for range of traits, selecting for deafness, and sex selection, and concludes that "The technical ability to provide these choices is not far from reality, but the ethical roadmap that will offer direction to physicians is not as clearly laid out."[57] In other words, the opinion does not attempt to lay out the ethical roadmap for these uses of PGD; it only notes that ethical dilemmas related to PGD will continue to arise and must be dealt with in due course.

A 2007 ACOG Ethics Committee Opinion on sex selection is more decisive. The document states conclusively that while the Committee "supports the practice of offering patients procedures for the purpose of preventing serious sex-linked diseases," it "opposes meeting requests for sex selection for personal and family reasons, including family balancing, because of the concern that such requests may ultimately support sexist practice." This opinion is not prefaced with the statement that it is not intended to prescribe a specific course of action, and its content, that ACOG opposes sex selection of any kind, is reiterated in the 2008 opinion on genetic testing.[58]

ACOG has published two additional documents that while not specifically on the various uses of PGD, mention PGD and characterize it in a particular way. A 2009 Committee on Genetics Opinion about

DOI: 10.1057/9781137515445.0006

preimplantation genetic screening (screening embryos for aneuploidy) compares PGS to PGD, which it says has become a "standard method of testing for single gene disorders" and has been "used for diagnosis of translocations and single-gene disorders, such as cystic fibrosis, X-linked recessive conditions, and inherited mutations, which increase one's risk of developing cancer."[59] Another ACOG Genetics Committee document similarly refers to PGD in terms of its medical applications. It describes PGD as a tool that can be used to identify "Single-gene disorders and chromosomal abnormalities, such as deletions and translocations" and notes that molecular testing (including PGD) can be employed "to determine whether an individual or fetus has inherited a disease-causing gene mutation."[60] While these documents do not preclude the use of PGD for nonmedical purposes, they focus on PGD's therapeutic capabilities.

ACOG holds strong views about the use of reproductive tools for sex selection, but otherwise does not indicate precisely when PGD ought to be used. Nevertheless, their documents imply that PGD is and should be primarily employed for medical purposes, though nonmedical applications other than sex selection are not prohibited or actively discouraged.

The American College of Medical Genetics has not published guidelines specifically on the use of PGD, but it does have a policy statement on prenatal and preconception screening. As with most of the ACOG documents, the statement opens with a disclaimer:

> ACMG position statements are developed primarily as educational resources for medical geneticists to help them provide quality clinical laboratory genetic services. Adherence to this statement is voluntary and does not necessarily ensure a successful medical outcome. This position statement should not be considered inclusive of all proper procedures and tests or exclusive of other procedures and tests that are reasonably directed to obtaining the same results. In determining the propriety of any specific procedure or test, the clinical laboratory geneticist should apply his or her own professional judgment to the specific circumstances presented by the individual patient or specimen…[61]

The content of the document states that there "There must be validated clinical association between the mutation(s) detected and the severity of the disorder." This may suggest that reproductive genetic testing should be used primarily for severe genetic disorders, but the opinion also notes that for "disorders with mild phenotypes, variable expression, low penetrance and/or" are "characterized by an adult onset," testing should be performed in a "transparent" fashion, "allowing patients to

DOI: 10.1057/9781137515445.0006

opt out of receiving these test results" if they wish.[62] It is unclear how these statements on carrier screening could be rendered applicable to PGD. Patients who request the use of PGD for milder conditions (or nonmedical conditions) would not choose to opt out of receiving the test results that they desire. It is therefore not apparent whether the ACMG would oppose or discourage the use of preimplantation genetic testing of embryos for less severe disorders.

Like ACOG, the ACMG seems to emphasize the use of reproductive genetic testing for medical purposes, but it has not published guidelines outlining how and when it believes PGD ought to be used. Thus none of the major professional societies relevant to the use of PGD have taken a strong stance to date, with the exception of ACOG on sex selection, on PGD's various applications. When discussing self-regulation in reproductive medical practice, it is necessary to view self-regulation not only as a theoretical solution to concerns with PGD, but also as a practical means of guiding the actions of medical professionals. The current approaches of the ASRM, ACOG, and ACMG toward regulating PGD or closely related techniques do not suggest that professional self-regulation will play a key role in limiting the use of PGD for nonmedical purposes in the near future.

Summary: the pros and cons of government regulation vs. professional self-regulation

Despite the limited nature of self-regulation regarding PGD at present, medical societies seem to feel strongly that regulation by medical professionals is preferable to state intervention. In 2006, two former ASRM presidents and the then current ASRM Executive Director published a paper specifically on the subject of professional self-regulation of PGD, in which they raised several serious objections to government regulation. In the piece, the authors argued that self-regulation was "more consistent with the U.S. government not funding ART" since in their opinion, "regulatory oversight should parallel funding."[63] Furthermore, they suggested that regulation by the state might result in poorly crafted laws, which could be worse than no regulation at all. As an example, they cited an instance in Texas in the 1990s when a bill intended to mandate coverage of infertility treatment "mutated into a bill in which carriers merely had to 'offer' coverage." The outcome was that "fewer citizens were served than before legislative action" because insurers offered prohibitively expensive supplemental coverage for infertility treatment. The authors also asserted that attempting to develop a list of conditions for which PGD should or should not be used would be "hopelessly naïve" because of the rate at which new gene products for various genes are being discovered. Adhering to a list of approved indications, they contended, "would exert a chilling effect" on research into the development of new tests, and such a list would "inevitably...not be updated in a timely fashion."

The objections to state regulation of PGD by the ASRM leadership are significant, but not necessarily decisive. It would be possible, for example, to design a regulatory system that was clear about the conditions for which PGD may not be used (e.g. sex selection or selection for a disability) and flexible or even open-ended regarding the conditions for which PGD could be used. This might ameliorate the chilling and delaying effect that the authors fear regarding the development of new tests and the approval of new conditions. Such regulation would also, at least theoretically, avoid the "bluntness" of regulation, in which it is difficult for individual patients with specific or rare conditions to access the treatment they need. Furthermore, there is no particular reason why regulation ought to parallel government funding, as long as society's interest in regulating a particular activity is sufficiently clear and legitimate. The concern with bad regulation, whether due to the unforeseen consequences of poor wording or moral legislation by state legislators who object to all or most uses of PGD, is an important concern. However, the possibility that regulation might go awry is not sufficient justification for not regulating PGD at all.

Another important factor to take into consideration is the real or perceived financial conflict of interest that physicians who recommend or carry out PGD may have. For example, in 2012, a number of popular media articles revealed that some fertility clinics have partnered with companies offering loans to patients in need of fertility treatment.[64] In these situations, there is clearly a potential conflict of interest for the physicians who both promote a fertility lender and prescribe treatment.[65] While there is no evidence regarding such conflicts of interest and the recommendation of PGD in particular, we must acknowledge the risk that professional associations might be reluctant to suggest banning or limiting services for which patients are willing to pay.

On the other hand, self-regulation by professional organizations has the significant advantage of drawing on the support of the medical practitioners who carry out PGD. The expertise of fertility specialists and medical geneticists, as well as their cooperation, is critical to the process of designing and implementing regulations on the use of PGD. If physicians can truly demonstrate that government regulation would hamper their ability to provide the best treatment possible to their patients, legislators should be wary of imposing regulations upon them. Furthermore, it is crucial that regulators heed the warnings of the ASRM regarding the potential for the regulation of PGD to go awry and make sure to involve physicians in the policy development process.

Regulatory flexibility in scientific and moral gray areas: the example of the HFEA

A primary concern raised by the ASRM leaders is that a list of PGD conditions could not be readily updated and would be overly restrictive. Another concern that we encountered in our conversations with bioethicists and physicians was with how the ethical decisions regarding what conditions to allow would be made; if the ASRM Ethics Committee could not agree about whether elective sex selection ought to be discouraged, how would a group of legislators be able to establish ethical norms, and which norms would be the right ones to establish? Some have suggested that the diversity of ethical opinions might be a reason not to regulate PGD.[66] The HFEA presents one model of regulating in the scientific and moral gray areas presented by PGD.

The HFEA allows PGD to be used for a given condition after a License Committee has approved its use, which follows an application process by a fertility clinic on behalf of a patient. The application requires that clinics demonstrate that the condition is serious and the risk is significant and includes a summary of papers and documents relevant to the case. The application is then sent to clinical geneticists in the UK for peer review and posted on the HFEA website for public consultation before it is considered by a License Committee.[67] In addition to the process for approving new conditions, there is a general ban on the use of PGD for sex selection for nonmedical purposes, and each use of PGD for HLA tissue matching must be approved on a case-by-case basis. To date, the HFEA has approved the use of PGD for 287 conditions.[68] Forty-eight of these conditions were approved in the year between April 1, 2012 and March 31, 2013 in fourteen separate License Committee meetings.[69] The

DOI: 10.1057/9781137515445.0006

HFEA also posts a list of conditions awaiting approval online and the public can email in comments about whether a given condition should be approved.

The work of an HFEA License Committee is clearly defined in the guidelines laid out in the Code of Practice for the approval of new conditions. The Code of Practice states that a license may be given for "Embryos that are known to have a gene, chromosome or mitochondrion abnormality involving a significant risk that a person with the abnormality will have or develop: a. a serious physical or mental disability; b. a serious illness, or; c. any other serious medical condition."[70] Essentially, License Committees must gauge how serious a disorder is, taking into account such issues as the views of the people seeking treatment, the likely degree of suffering associated with the condition, the availability of effective therapy, the speed of degeneration in a progressive disorder, the extent of any intellectual impairment, and the extent of social support available.[71]

For certain categories of conditions, such as lower penetrance and later onset conditions, the HFEA has conducted wider policy reviews that included consultations with the public. For example, the HFEA conducted a review of the use of PGD for lower penetrance inherited cancer conditions that involved an open meeting and a written document to which stakeholders were invited to send responses.[72] The reviewing committee also sought out the views of people who were at risk of developing lower penetrance inherited cancers in order to ensure that their perspectives were considered.[73]

In practice, the process can take anywhere from two to six months from the time an application is submitted to the time the condition is approved. It is rare that the HFEA denies approval, though it may take longer for lower penetrance conditions with variable phenotypes to be approved. Many clinics wait until after the condition has been approved to develop a genetic test, since developing tests is expensive. In total, therefore, it can take 12 to 15 months for a couple to carry out PGD from when they first arrive at a clinic.[74]

The HFEA thus responds to changes in the science surrounding PGD and the development of tests for new conditions with a rolling approval process. In response to the difficulty of deciding acceptable and unacceptable uses in an ethical gray area, the HFEA attempts to draw upon the views of a range of relevant stakeholders before reaching its conclusions.[75] In addition to the opinions of patients, clinical geneticists,

DOI: 10.1057/9781137515445.0006

and the general public, the HFEA considers the recommendations of its Ethics and Law Committee, which is comprised of doctors, lawyers, and philosophers. While the HFEA model requires couples to wait 12–15 months before carrying out PGD for new conditions, the large number of already approved uses of PGD, which include late onset and lower penetrance conditions in addition to the archetypal severe early onset diseases, will cover most cases.[76] This model can therefore serve as an example of how PGD can be regulated in a way that combines flexibility in the approval of new conditions with strict rules regarding sex selection and other nonmedical uses of PGD.

Who should decide?

In many ways, the question of whether and how to regulate PGD is about whose opinions ought to be taken into consideration and how much weight they should be given. Should elected officials, fertility specialists, families, or the general public decide what uses of PGD to allow? Each group contributes its own hopes and fears—from the freedom to make one's own reproductive choices to the ability to care for one's patients without intervention to deeply held convictions about what uses of technology are ethical and just. Correspondingly, each group has reason to believe that its views should be heeded, and in some cases given more weight than others.

There are some limited data on the views of fertility specialists versus the general public regarding the regulation of PGD. A 2004 survey of fertility clinic directors administered by the Genetics and Public Policy Center revealed that 95% of the directors agreed or strongly agreed that professional societies are "best suited to create standards and guidelines relating to PGD."[77] This did not mean that the clinic directors were necessarily content with the state of self-regulation at the time or believed that it was sustainable in the long term; 43% of directors believed PGD raised ethical "questions or sensibilities" and 85% of directors agreed or strongly agreed that PGD would become "more standardized across clinics and laboratories because of stronger practice guidelines." It would be interesting to examine if these opinions have changed over the past ten years. However, given the disclaimers in the statements released by the relevant professional societies in the intervening time, and the fact that the position of the ASRM Ethics Committee on sex selection (the

DOI: 10.1057/9781137515445.0006

most common nonmedical use of PGD) has become weaker, rather than stronger, it is unlikely that opinions on this matter have shifted radically.

By contrast, a sample of 4,843 Americans surveyed in 2004 indicated that 20% believed PGD should be banned, 24% supported government regulation for safety and quality, 37% supported government regulation for safety, quality, and ethics, and 17% supported no government regulation.[78] Thus a substantial majority of those surveyed favored some kind of government involvement in the regulation of PGD, and the largest section believed that the government ought to play a role in regulating the morality of PGD usage. It is likely, however, that most Americans would not have a nuanced understanding of the benefits and shortcomings of self-regulation by professional organizations and some may believe that government involvement is necessary for any regulation to occur. The researchers also noted that those who supported government regulation of PGD's ethics had a variety of views about what uses are ethically acceptable. Nonetheless, the 2004 surveys clearly demonstrate a divergence between the views of the general public and medical professionals in infertility on whether the government should participate in the regulation of PGD.

An exploration of the question of how to weigh these differing views, as well as the views of other groups, is beyond the scope of this book, as it approaches complex issues of democratic theory and the nature and process of democratic deliberation. Such an exploration would be essential to formulating PGD policy and designing appropriate regulatory mechanisms. The example of the HFEA described here presents one model for taking account of the views of multiple stakeholders in designing regulations. It is therefore unnecessary for disagreement about ethics and the role of government to serve as an insurmountable obstacle to the regulation of PGD.

The bottom line

Ultimately, the answer to the question "should PGD be more regulated?" depends on whether or not one believes that the present state of self-regulation is sufficient, which will in turn depend on one's views regarding government involvement in medical practice, reproductive autonomy, and whether or not current uses of PGD are morally troubling. If, for

DOI: 10.1057/9781137515445.0006

example, you believe that sex selection is more ethically problematic than the limitation of patients' reproductive choices regarding the sex of their child and the intervention of the government into doctor–patient relations, you will likely support government regulation to restrict access to PGD for elective sex selection.[79] In the future, as more genes for nonmedical (and medical) conditions are discovered, the issue of regulation will become more pressing. If professional societies do not develop more definitive, stronger guidelines for medical practitioners (and perhaps even if they do), government regulation will become more necessary and more likely.

Notes

1   Robertson, John. "Assisting Reproduction, Choosing Genes and the Scope of Reproductive Autonomy." *The George Washington Law Review* 76.6 (2008): 1490–1513.

2   Ibid.

3   Buck v. Bell, 274 U.S. 200 (1927).

4   Leslie-Miller, Jana. "From Buck to Bell: Responsible Reproduction in the Twentieth Century." *Maryland Journal of Contemporary Legal Issues* 123.8 (1997): 123–150.

5   Skinner v. Oklahoma, 316 U.S. 535 (1942).

6   Griswold v. Connecticut, 381 U.S. 479, 480 (1965).

7   Roe v. Wade, 410 U.S. 113 (1973).

8   Ibid.

9   Robertson, John. "Assisting Reproduction, Choosing Genes and the Scope of Reproductive Autonomy."

10   Ibid.

11   Granted, quality of life determinations are not entirely divorced from social and cultural context. How we determine quality of life, in terms of opportunities available, health, socioeconomic status, and other factors is itself a product of a particular society, and thus it may be impossible to make quality of life determinations in an entirely "objective" manner. We have already acknowledged that all conceptions of disability or disease will inevitably incorporate some social biases. Nevertheless, there is some merit in making an effort to compare populations on the basis of socioeconomic or educational standards. Though imperfect, measuring certain categories that we perceive as important to well-being is preferable to making judgments based on rationales such as "I wouldn't want to live like that" or worse, "I'd rather die than live like that." Furthermore, at least quality of life

measurements are not specific to a particular condition and can be applied consistently across different populations.

12   Scott, Rosamund. *Choosing between Possible Lives.* Page 215.
13   Colls, P. *et al.* (2009) "Preimplantation Genetic Diagnosis for Gender Selection in the USA."
14   Ibid.
15   Berkowitz, Jonathan M. and Jack W. Snyder. "Racism and Sexism in Medically Assisted Conception." *Bioethics* 12.1 (1998): 25–44.
16   Buchanan, Allen E., Dan W. Brock, Norman Daniels, and Daniel Wikler. *From Chance to Choice: Genetics and Justice.* Page 13.
17   Wilson, Robert. "Environmental Regulation of the Human Gene Pool as a Genetic Commons." *N.Y.U. Environmental Law Journal* 5 (1996): 833–857.
18   Darnovsky, Marcy. "A Slippery Slope to Human Germline Modification." *Nature* 499.7457 (2013): 127.
19   Wilkinson, Stephen. *Choosing Tomorrow's Children: The Ethics of Selective Reproduction.* Page 24.
20   Ibid. Page 152.
21   Lombardo, Paul A. *Three Generations, No Imbeciles: Eugenics, the Supreme Court, and Buck v. Bell.* Baltimore: Johns Hopkins University Press, 2008.
22   Ibid. Page 158.
23   Galton, Francis. "Eugenics: Its Definition, Scope, and Aims." *American Journal of Sociology* 10.1 (1904): 1–25.
24   Unlike coercive eugenics, laissez-faire eugenics is not coercive, at least in the physical sense, and does not restrict reproductive autonomy, but can be criticized on the grounds that it instills and perpetuates the view that some people are genetically better or worse.
25   Wilkinson, Stephen. *Choosing Tomorrow's Children: The Ethics of Selective Reproduction.* Page 156.
26   Baruch, Susannah. "PGD: Genetic Testing of Embryos in the United States."
27   Malek and Daar (2012) argue for such a legal obligation to select against very severe disorders when a couple is already undergoing IVF and PGD, although they would not consider dwarfism to be a sufficiently serious condition to warrant the use of state force. It is unclear, however, when such a law would be useful, since parents already undergoing IVF and PGD would likely be doing so precisely in order to select against the severe disease.
28   The concept of coercion is complex and cannot be fully discussed here. It is possible, for example, for someone to be coerced into *not* performing a specific action; coercion is not limited to forcing people to do things. Furthermore, many uses of state power can be considered coercive in a certain sense. In this section, however, we use "coercion" to refer to the use of state power to force people to select a certain embryo over another, as this is the focus of the criterion regarding the means used by authoritarian

DOI: 10.1057/9781137515445.0006

eugenics. On the ethical assessment of coercion generally, see Gaylin, Willard and Bruce Jennings, *The Perversion of Autonomy: Coercion and Constraints in a Liberal Society*, 2nd ed., Washington, DC: Georgetown University Press, 2004.

29   Until recently, Italy had such a ban of PGD, but has recently begun to allow its use for a set of limited conditions. See Gianaroli, Luca, Anna Maria Crivello, Ilaria Stanghellini, Anna Pia Ferraretti, Carla Tabanelli, and Maria Cristina Magli. "Reiterative Changes in the Italian Regulation on IVF: The Effect on PGD Patients' Reproductive Decisions." *Reproductive BioMedicine Online* 28.1 (2013): 125–132.

30   Baruch S., G. Javitt, J. Scott, and K. Hudson. *Preimplantation Genetic Diagnosis: A Discussion of Challenges, Concerns, and Preliminary Policy Options Related to the Genetic Testing of Human Embryos*. Washington, DC: Genetics and Public Policy Center, 2004.

31   Murray, Thomas H., "Stirring the Simmering 'Designer Baby' Pot," *Science* 343 (March 14, 2014): 1208–1210.

32   Those who object to the disposal of embryos known to be carrying harmful hereditary conditions would also have to object to the disposal of healthy embryos, which takes place during IVF if couples do not choose to donate their embryos to other couples or to research (embryos donated for research purposes are also destroyed). Thus while some find the disposal of embryos with "unwanted" genes particularly unpalatable, this practice does not necessarily actually introduce an additional complication.

33   Gutierrez, Alberto. "Warning Letter to 23andMe, Inc." *Inspections, Compliance, Enforcement, and Criminal Investigations*. Food and Drug Administration, November 22, 2013. Web. March 14, 2014.

34   Baruch S. *et al.* (2004) *Reproductive Genetic Testing: Issues and Options for Policymakers.*

35   The FDA indicated in July 2014 that it will begin to regulate the safety and efficacy of laboratory-developed tests (LDTs), including many genetic tests, although it remains uncertain precisely what the final guidelines will entail, and how "safety and efficacy" will be determined. Based on the draft guidance released on September 30, 2014, it appears that the FDA will largely rely on published scientific data in order to ensure that LDTs are accurate and produce clinically valid results (*Anticipated Details of the Draft Guidance for Industry, Food and Drug Administration Staff, and Clinical Laboratories.* Working paper. Silver Spring, MD: FDA, 2014.). Nonetheless, the FDA will still not be able to regulate under what circumstances a physician can order a genetic test.

36   Stankovic, Bratislav. " 'It's a Designer Baby!'—Opinions on Regulation of Preimplantation Genetic Diagnosis." *UCLA Journal of Law and Technology* 3 (2005): n. pag.

DOI: 10.1057/9781137515445.0006

37 "Vaccines, Blood & Biologics." *Tissue & Tissue Products*. Food and Drug Administration, n.d. Web. March 14, 2014. <http://www.fda.gov/biologicsbloodvaccines/tissuetissueproducts/default.htm>; Baruch S. *et al.* (2004) *Reproductive Genetic Testing: Issues and Options for Policymakers.*

38 "Vaccines, Blood & Biologics: Compliance Program Guidance Manual." *Tissue & Tissue Products*. Food and Drug Administration, n.d. Web. March 14, 2014.

39 Stankovic, B. " 'It's a Designer Baby!'—Opinions on Regulation of Preimplantation Genetic Diagnosis."

40 *2012 ART Fertility Clinic Success Rates Report.* Rep.: Centers for Disease Control and Prevention, 2014.

41 Yost, Judith. *CLIA and Genetic Testing Oversight.* Rep.: Center for Medicare and Medicaid Services, 2008.

42 "The Fertility Clinic Success Rate and Certification Act." *Policy Documents.* Centers for Disease Control and Prevention, October 31, 2013. Web. April 8, 2014. <http://www.cdc.gov/art/Policy.htm>.

43 "ASRM/CAP Reproductive Laboratory Accreditation Program." *ASRM Annual Meeting: ASRM/CAP Reproductive Laboratory Accreditation Program Inspector Training Seminar.* N.p., n.d. Web. April 9, 2014. <https://www.asrm.org/ASRM2013_CAP_Course/>.

44 *HFEA Standing Orders.* Rep.: Human Fertilisation and Embryology Authority, 2013.

45 Baruch S. *et al.* (2004) *Reproductive Genetic Testing: Issues and Options for Policymakers.*

46 Ibid.

47 Ibid.

48 Fossett, James W., Alicia R. Ouellette, Sean Philpott, David Magnus, and Glenn McGee. "Federalism and Bioethics: States and Moral Pluralism." *Hastings Center Report* 37.6 (2007): 24–35.

49 Committee on Health Care for Underserved Women of the American Congress of Obstetricians and Gynecologists. "Abortion Access and Training: Committee Opinion." Number 424, January 2009.

50 Saad, Lydia. "Americans' Abortion Views Steady Amid Gosnell Trial." Gallup.com, May 10, 2013. Web. March 17, 2014.

51 Murray, Thomas H., "Stirring the Simmering 'Designer Baby' Pot," *Science* 343 (March 14, 2014): 1208–1210.

52 Ethics Committee of the American Society for Reproductive Medicine. "Sex Selection and Preimplantation Genetic Diagnosis." *Fertility and Sterility* 72.4 (1999): 595–598.

53 Ethics Committee of the American Society for Reproductive Medicine. "Preconception Gender Selection for Nonmedical Reasons": 861–864.

54 Pers. comm. Dr Paula Amato, Chair, Ethics Committee of the American Society for Reproductive Medicine, January 16, 2014.

DOI: 10.1057/9781137515445.0006

55   Practice Committee of the American Society for Reproductive Medicine. "Preimplantation Genetic Testing: A Practice Committee Opinion": 136–143.

56   Ethics Committee of the American Society for Reproductive Medicine. "Use of Preimplantation Genetic Diagnosis for Serious Adult Onset Conditions: A Committee Opinion": 54–57.

57   Committees on Ethics and Genetics of the American Congress of Obstetricians and Gynecologists. "Ethical Issues in Genetic Testing." Number 410, June 2008.

58   Committee on Ethics of the American Congress of Obstetricians and Gynecologists. "Sex Selection." Number 360, February 2007.

59   Committee on Genetics of the American Congress of Obstetricians and Gynecologists. "Preimplantation Genetic Screening for Aneuploidy." Number 430, March 2009.

60   Committee on Genetics of the American Congress of Obstetricians and Gynecologists. "Technology Assessment: Genetics and Molecular Diagnostic Testing." Number 11, February 2014.

61   Grody, Wayne, Barry H. Thompson, Anthony R. Gregg, Lora H. Bean, Kristin G. Monaghan, Adele Schneider, and Roger V. Lebo. "ACMG Position Statement on Prenatal/Preconception Expanded Carrier Screening." American College of Medical Genetics and Genomics. *Genetics in Medicine* 15.5 (2013): 482–483.

62   Ibid.

63   Simpson, Joe, Robert Rebar, and Sandra Carson. "Professional Self-Regulation for Preimplantation Genetic Diagnosis: Experience of the American Society for Reproductive Medicine and Other Professional Societies." *Fertility and Sterility* 85 (2006): 1653–1660.

64   See, for example, Ubel, Peter. "Are Infertility Doctors Turning into Predatory Bankers?" *Forbes.* Forbes Magazine, December 11, 2012. Web. September 22, 2014. <http://www.forbes.com/sites/peterubel/2012/12/11/are-infertility-doctors-turning-into-predatory-bankers/>.

65   Von Hagel, Alison. "Banking on Infertility: Medical Ethics and the Marketing of Fertility Loans." *Hastings Center Report* 43.6 (2013): 15–17.

66   Pers. comm. Prof. Anita Silvers, Chair of Philosophy at San Francisco State University, February 8, 2014.

67   Pers. comm. Ms Alison Lashwood, Clinical Lead in PGD, Centre for Preimplantation Genetic Diagnosis, Guy's and St Thomas' Hospital, London, UK. March 26, 2014.

68   "PGD Conditions Licensed by the HFEA." *Your Treatment and Storage Options.* Human Fertilisation and Embryology Authority, n.d. Web. March 22, 2014.

69   *New PGD Conditions Licensed by the HFEA between 1 April 2012 and 31 March 2013.* Rep. N.p.: Human Fertilisation and Embryology Authority, 2013.

DOI: 10.1057/9781137515445.0006

70   *Human Fertilisation and Embryology Act (as amended).* Schedule 2. London, United Kingdom, 1990.

71   "Clinical Decision-Making." *HFEA Guidance on Preimplantation Genetic Testing.* Human Fertilisation and Embryology Authority, 2006.

72   *Choices and Boundaries: A Summary of Responses to the HFEA Public Discussion.* Rep.: Human Fertilisation and Embryology Authority, 2006.

73   Ibid.

74   Pers. comm. Ms Alison Lashwood, Clinical Lead in PGD, Centre for Preimplantation Genetic Diagnosis, Guy's and St Thomas' Hospital, London, UK. March 26, 2014. Ms Lashwood noted that this timeframe might be slightly different for other centers, as the analysis can be done in different ways.

75   *Authority Decision on the Use of PGD for Lower Penetrance, Later Onset Inherited Disorders.* Rep.: Human Fertilisation and Embryology Authority, 2006.

76   Ms Lashwood estimated that 80% of referrals for PGD are covered by already approved conditions.

77   Baruch, S. *et al.* (2008) "Genetic Testing of Embryos: Practices and Perspectives of US in Vitro Fertilization Clinics."

78   Hudson, K. (2006) "Preimplantation Genetic Diagnosis: Public Policy and Public Attitudes."

79   Political theory would also be useful in weighing the different values at stake in the decision of whether and how to regulate PGD. For example, a libertarian liberal would likely prioritize individual rights to procreative autonomy over the other considerations, unless the rights of individual future children were seen as being at risk. An egalitarian liberal might be especially concerned with the problem of unequal access to PGD. A communitarian may be particularly troubled by the expressivist problem with selection against disabilities and the prospect of elective sex selection reinforcing harmful gender stereotypes. In future work, it would be helpful to elucidate the relationships between different political philosophies and the various approaches to PGD regulation.

DOI: 10.1057/9781137515445.0006

5

Paying for PGD

Abstract: *In the final chapter, we summarize the challenges that couples around the United States face when attempting to finance PGD, along with the factors that insurance companies consider when deciding whether to offer coverage for PGD and for what purposes. The chapter ends with a brief recapitulation of the major conclusions of the essay and several avenues for future research.*

Bayefsky, Michelle and Bruce Jennings. *Regulating Preimplantation Genetic Diagnosis in the United States: The Limits of Unlimited Selection.* New York: Palgrave Macmillan, 2015. DOI: 10.1057/9781137515445.0007.

Regulatory structures often mirror payment structures.[1] This makes sense; if the government is going to pay for a procedure, it must determine what uses it should cover. Though funding a limited set of applications does not preclude other privately funded uses, government funding creates the need for at least some regulation or consideration of what applications of a particular procedure should be seen as necessary or acceptable.

Since carrying out PGD requires couples to undergo IVF beforehand, and IVF costs about $12,000 per cycle while PGD costs $3,550, payment for IVF is a major issue for those seeking to carry out PGD.[2] Unfortunately, IVF is typically not covered by insurance plans. In fact, it is extremely unlikely that an insurance plan would cover IVF unless one happened to live in one of the seven states where insurance companies are required by law to cover at least one cycle of IVF.[3] Of the fifteen states mentioned in the introduction that have laws relating to infertility coverage, three specifically exclude coverage for IVF (New York, California, and Louisiana), two allow insurance companies to exclude IVF (Texas and Ohio), three do not clearly define infertility or specify what treatments must be covered (Rhode Island, West Virginia, and Montana), and seven require some amount of coverage for IVF (Arkansas, Connecticut, Hawaii, Illinois, Maryland, Massachusetts, and New Jersey). In these seven states, coverage ranges from one cycle of IVF (in Hawaii, where "infertility" is defined as trying unsuccessfully to have a child for five years) to unlimited coverage for fertility services, including IVF, in Massachusetts.[4] In the other 43 states, insurance coverage for IVF is not required and if it were offered at all, would likely be part of an expensive insurance package.

Some major health insurance companies do, however, provide coverage for PGD. United Healthcare, for example, includes coverage of PGD "for the diagnosis of known genetic disorders" under their medical benefit, unless there are specific exclusions in a particular plan.[5] Aetna also offers PGD coverage and considers PGD medically necessary "when there is a need to diagnose specific, detectable single gene mutations."[6] The Aetna policy notes, however, that the IVF procedure is covered only for persons "with ART benefits who meet medical necessity criteria for IVF."[7] In other words, the woman or couple must be diagnosed with infertility, which, depending on age, would involve proof that less invasive interventions had been unsuccessful or a diagnosis of tubal factor infertility.[8] Most couples in need of PGD to prevent passing on a

DOI: 10.1057/9781137515445.0007

heritable condition would not meet these criteria, and thus even if they were in a state that mandates IVF coverage or happen to have an Aetna plan that includes IVF, their IVF would not be covered. Some fertility specialists will sign off on a diagnosis of infertility for patients in need of PGD even if they do not technically meet the criteria. They might, for instance, allow couples to claim that they have tried to have a child for the requisite period of time in order to qualify for fertility treatment.[9] For a plan that requires couples to undergo less invasive treatment before utilizing IVF, though, it would be difficult to claim that those treatments had been carried out. Another major carrier, Cigna health insurance, also covers medically necessary PGD but not IVF, unless the patient's plan specifically covers IVF.[10]

Overall, it is difficult to determine how many people have insurance coverage that would fund PGD. While some of the major companies offer plans that cover PGD in order to select against genes that cause serious disease, it is unclear how common these plans are or whether coverage is primarily limited to obscure and expensive supplemental plans. There is no comprehensive database that tracks the specific benefits covered by insurance plans across America. On fertility advice websites and chat rooms, there are many complaints about the lack of coverage for PGD, so it seems as though PGD coverage is not common despite the policies that can be found online.[11]

From a business perspective, it is not immediately apparent why health insurance companies do not make a more concerted effort to ensure that IVF and PGD are used to prevent the birth of children with serious genetic conditions. Now that people with preexisting conditions cannot be excluded from health insurance plans, insurance companies are required to cover expensive treatments for children with serious heritable illnesses. Would it not be better to help parents avoid having such children to begin with? A senior official at a large health benefit company, who was interviewed for this book, outlined three major considerations that prevented insurance companies from offering coverage for IVF and PGD despite the financial incentive to prevent the birth of seriously diseased and disabled children.[12]

First, it is not feasible from a public relations standpoint for insurance companies to cover IVF for patients who need PGD and not for patients with fertility issues unrelated to passing on genetic disease. Health insurance companies, which our informant noted are already not very popular among the public, cannot be seen as assigning monetary values to

DOI: 10.1057/9781137515445.0007

lives with different kinds of diseases and using the targeted availability of insurance coverage to prevent the birth of people with particular conditions. Covering IVF only for people who need PGD is not an option, then, and IVF is too expensive for insurance companies to want to cover the procedure for every infertile person who could benefit from its use. Especially now that health insurance companies cannot turn down applicants with preexisting conditions, no company can afford to be the first in a state that offers coverage of IVF at a reasonable cost, because then everyone who knows he or she needs IVF will purchase that plan. This is the problem of adverse selection, which can only be solved with a mandate like the ones implemented in the seven states listed. If all plans in a state must include coverage of IVF, then insurance companies can cover IVF for patients who need PGD to prevent passing on a serious genetic disease along with the patients who need IVF for other fertility issues.

Aside from the public policy concern, another potential difficulty with paying for IVF only for those who need PGD is that the Genetic Information Nondiscrimination Act (GINA) forbids health insurance companies from discriminating against customers on the basis on genetic information. The senior official we interviewed suggested that *not paying* for IVF for people *without* genetic conditions could be construed as discrimination. However, GINA specifically states that insurance companies cannot use genetic information to discriminate regarding "premium or contribution amounts" but that this rule should not "be construed to preclude a group health plan...from obtaining and using the results of a genetic test in making a determination regarding payment."[13] Insurance companies are allowed to decide what treatments to cover on the basis of genetic testing; they just cannot use test results to raise premiums for people who test positive for disease-related genes. Thus it would probably not be considered discriminatory to pay for a particular procedure for someone with a genetic condition and not for those without such a condition.

A final reason insurance companies might not go out of their way to cover IVF for those who need PGD is that people frequently switch insurance plans, so it may not be worth it for a company to pay for IVF and PGD in order to avoid having a child with a serious genetic condition on their rolls. Perhaps if it could be demonstrated that the children who would not have been born if PGD had been more accessible became a financial burden to a particular company, it would be in that company's best interest to pay for IVF and PGD for that family. However, no such data are available, and it is hard to imagine that it will be possible to collect the information necessary to make this kind of analysis.

Gaining greater coverage for fertility treatment for those in need of PGD seems to be an uphill battle. In addition to the reluctance of insurance companies due to the costs of IVF, some medical professionals believe that state mandates for IVF coverage are a bad idea. For example, in the paper by ASRM leaders on self-regulation and PGD, the authors wrote:

> Legislation forcing insurance carriers to cover ART or PGD is not, however, synonymous with governmental funding; in a mandated insurance program, individual citizens or their employers pay, not the government. Onerous restriction or oversight through unfunded mandates will inevitably result in lack of service. Premiums will inevitably increase, making full-time employees with health benefits prohibitively expensive to employers. Unfunded mandates may appear to be a tempting short-term solution, but they actually constitute a recipe for unpredictable mischief. Until the United States or individual states fully fund ART and PGD, mandates should be restricted to creation of registries, accreditation of labs, and credentialing of professionals.[14]

It seems unlikely, however, that mandating that insurance plans fund a cycle or two of IVF would singlehandedly make health benefits prohibitively expensive to employers. In 2012, about 1.5% of births in America were the result of IVF.[15] While this is not an insignificant figure, coverage for IVF would probably not make the difference between health insurance being affordable or unaffordable. Furthermore, it is unclear why fertility specialists in particular would oppose state mandates for coverage. Even if the mandate were only a short-term fix, more of their patients would be able to afford the IVF treatment they need to have a child.[16]

Even for advocates for insurance mandates for IVF coverage, such as those at RESOLVE, the national infertility association, expanding access to IVF for patients who need PGD does not constitute a major focus of their work. RESOLVE's mission is to improve the lives of people with infertility, which is not treated as a disease like any other. According to RESOLVE President and CEO Barbara Collura, while the organization's work at the state and federal levels aims to preserve and increase access to infertility treatment for all those who need it, increasing access specifically for patients who require PGD "has not come up as a legislative issue required their focus." The organization's main goal is to

DOI: 10.1057/9781137515445.0007

convince state and national legislators that infertility is in fact a disease, and that its treatment ought to be covered by insurance. But Ms Collura added that state mandates provide limited coverage and that RESOLVE does not anticipate any new state mandates than the current fifteen.[17] Even if additional state mandates are passed, it is not guaranteed that patients who need PGD would be able to access IVF, since they are not technically infertile. However, it may be in insurance companies' best interest to fund IVF for those who need PGD if they are already required to pay for IVF for other patients with fertility problems. Thus, indirectly, work to increase the number of states with IVF mandates could benefit patients who need to use PGD to prevent transmitting a serious heritable disorder.

In this chapter, we have focused on payment for PGD for serious or severe conditions because insurance companies would not cover the use of PGD for purposes that were not considered medically necessary. Like the HFEA, insurance companies must consider what uses of PGD are sufficiently serious to warrant funding. They do not make these calculations based on which diseases are most expensive to treat if a child with the condition is born. Rather, once a benefit committee has decided to offer coverage for a particular procedure, a separate policy committee composed primarily of doctors in the field determines what it believes standard medical practice has deemed medically necessary.[18] For example, Anthem's PGD policy defines "medically necessary" as follows:

a. There have been three prior failed attempts at IVF
b. One of the partners is known to harbor a balanced translocation
c. Any of the first set of criteria and all of the second set of criteria are met:
   1. Set one:
      – Both partners are known carriers of the same autosomal recessive disorder
      – One partner is a known carrier of an autosomal recessive disorder, and the couple have previously produced offspring affected by that disorder
      – One partner is a known carrier of a single gene autosomal dominant disorder
      – One partner is a known carrier of a single gene X-linked disorder

DOI: 10.1057/9781137515445.0007

2. Set two:
   - A specific mutation, or set of mutations, has been identified, that specifically identifies the genetic disorder with a high degree of reliability
   - The genetic disorder is associated with severe disability or has a lethal natural history
   - Testing is accompanied by genetic counseling.
d. When there is a documented history of an X-linked disorder, such that deselection of an affected embryo can be made on the basis of sex alone.
e. In families with a child with a bone marrow disorder requiring a stem cell transplant, and in whom there is no other source of a compatible bone marrow donor other than an HLA matched sibling.[19]

The rationale behind the Anthem PGD policy has been published online. The policy committee noted that evaluating "each specific genetic test for each abnormality is beyond the scope of this document," but "in general, in order to assure adequate sensitivity and specificity for the genetic test guiding the embryo deselection process, the genetic defect must be well characterized." The genes must be detectable, there must be "an understanding of the clinical significance of each mutation," and the severity of a genetic disorder must be considered as well. Since the committee did not compile a list of serious conditions, they decided that specific selection criteria would be treated on a case-by-case basis.[20]

The work of the Anthem's policy committee, then, was not very different from that of the HFEA's license committees. If everyone obtained funding for IVF and PGD after approval by an insurance company following the guidelines set by such a committee, it would be possible to regulate the use of PGD at the health insurance level. However, as discussed, insurance coverage for IVF and PGD is limited and people can always opt to pay out of pocket if they wish to avoid the rules set by an insurance policy committee. Anyone who desires to use PGD for purposes other than those considered "medically necessary," including sex selection or selection for a disability, would therefore not be constrained by what insurance companies have decided to cover.

DOI: 10.1057/9781137515445.0007

Conclusion

In this book, we have presented the major ethical, political, and economic considerations surrounding the regulation of preimplantation genetic diagnosis. PGD touches upon subjects that are fundamental to American society and culture: the nature of democratic decision-making, the limits of reproductive liberty, the way in which we view disabilities, and many other issues. Ultimately, PGD will only be regulated if Americans are sufficiently concerned with its ethical ramifications and if limiting reproductive autonomy and interfering with medical practice is deemed politically feasible. It will also be easier to regulate PGD if the government becomes more invested in directly funding medical services; medical professionals and patients may be more inclined to accept government oversight if it is coupled with greater access to the technology. Furthermore, as reproductive medicine and genetics continue to advance, allowing parents to test for more disease-related and other traits in their children, it is likely that calls to regulate PGD will become louder, more frequent, and more effective.

At the moment, the current absence of regulation is at odds with the opinions of the American public and the views of reproductive medical professionals. While opinion surveys on the use and regulation of PGD are now ten years old, the 2004 Genetic and Public Policy Center data indicated that both physicians and the general public believed there should be more regulation of PGD. Nearly all physicians felt this regulation should be self-directed, while a large segment of the public thought that the government should intervene to address both practical and ethical concerns. Nevertheless, a lack of sufficient public interest in the regulation of PGD and disagreement about the role of government in medical practice seem to hinder the development of regulation. Until a crisis situation arises, regulating PGD will probably not become a legislative priority despite the strong views that Americans seem to hold when asked about the ethics surrounding PGD.

It seems strange that there is not greater public interest in the use of PGD for nonmedical purposes. After all, there are public outcries about procedures like mitochondrial donation and therapeutic cloning because some worry they might lead to the creation of "designer babies." Meanwhile, the technology that currently affords parents selective capacity regarding their children's genes is unregulated.

DOI: 10.1057/9781137515445.0007

At the same time, we should be wary of slippery slope arguments about designer babies that reject, rather than moderate, advances in reproductive medicine and stray into the realm of science fiction instead of corresponding to scientific fact. Discussing the appropriate usage of PGD can be challenging to bioethicists, who must communicate medical advances to the public, along with the associated ethical implications, without creating undue fear or hype about potential abuses of reproductive technology. Especially in the United States, where embryo politics and reproductive rights are hotly contested, bioethicists must be careful to raise awareness of the ethical concerns related to certain uses of PGD without creating unnecessary controversy. After all, it is conceivable that state legislators might attempt to ban the use of PGD altogether. (Remember that 20% of those who responded to the 2004 survey believed PGD should be banned.) In some ways, focus on the ethical issues surrounding PGD may add fuel to a slowly burning fire that could end in rash legislative action.

Nevertheless, it has been the goal of this book to place concerns about the use of PGD in their proper ethical and scientific context and to highlight the political and economic hurdles that must be overcome in order for PGD regulation to be developed and implemented. We have concluded that government regulation has its drawbacks, but self-regulation also has considerable limitations. One possible compromise might be that if placed under pressure by impending government regulation, medical societies were to issue more definitive guidelines on the use of PGD. Stricter self-regulation would have the advantages of relying on the support of the relevant medical professionals and avoiding concerns about poorly crafted legislation impeding patient care. However, the rules would still not be legally binding and thus would not necessarily eliminate the uses of PGD that were considered unacceptable.

Future research in this area could focus on updating empirical data on the public's and medical professionals' views regarding the use and regulation of PGD. It would also be helpful to analyze the tradeoff between reproductive liberty and PGD regulation in greater depth, drawing on the work of political and constitutional theorists. A more thorough discussion of the nature of democratic deliberation and rulemaking in a diverse, pluralistic society would likewise contribute to our understanding of how PGD could and should be regulated in the United States.

It is too easy to resist regulating the use of PGD because of fear of controversy or resistance to change. While the question of how to

DOI: 10.1057/9781137515445.0007

legislate in a contentious area is difficult, it is not in itself a reason to avoid regulating PGD. If we ultimately decide not to regulate the use of PGD, it should be because we have considered the benefits and draw-backs of the various regulatory approaches and concluded that the status quo is the best option given the selective capacity available at present and in the near future. It should not be because we shied away from address-ing a controversial topic or asking probing questions about whether and when self-regulation by medical societies is appropriate. In the future, as genetic and reproductive technologies develop, we expect the regulation of PGD to be more widely discussed. When that time comes, we hope that this work can serve as a guide for those seeking to understand the ethical, political, and economic aspects of regulating PGD in the United States.

Notes

1   Simpson, Joe, Robert Rebar, and Sandra Carson. "Professional Self-Regulation for Preimplantation Genetic Diagnosis: Experience of the American Society for Reproductive Medicine and Other Professional Societies": 1653–1660.

2   "The Costs of Infertility Treatment." (2014) *RESOLVE: The National Infertility Association.*

3   "State Laws Related to Insurance Coverage for Infertility Treatment." (2014) National Conference of State Legislatures.

4   Ibid.

5   *Infertility Coverage Determination Guideline.* United Healthcare. May 1, 2013.

6   "Invasive Prenatal Diagnosis of Genetic Diseases." *Clinical Policy Bulletin.* Aetna, April 29, 2014. Web. September 19, 2014.

7   Ibid.

8   "Infertility." *Clinical Policy Bulletin.* Aetna, February 7, 2014. Web. March 30, 2014.

9   Pers. comm. Dr Mark Hughes, Founder and Director of Genesis Genetics, January 15, 2014.

10   *Cigna Medical Coverage Policy Preimplantation Genetic Diagnosis.* Cigna. October 15, 2013.

11   See, for example, "Preimplantation Genetic Diagnosis, Testing, and Screening Information and FAQ's." *PGD.* IVF1.com, November 3, 2013. Web. March 30, 2014.

12   Pers. comm. senior official of large health benefit company. February 19, 2014. This individual was interviewed on condition of anonymity.

DOI: 10.1057/9781137515445.0007

13   Genetic Information Nondiscrimination Act of 2008. H.R. 493, 110 Cong., Congressional Record (2008) (enacted).

14   Simpson, J. *et al.* "Professional Self-Regulation for Preimplantation Genetic Diagnosis: Experience of the American Society for Reproductive Medicine and Other Professional Societies."

15   Christensen, Jen. "Record Number of Women Using IVF to Get Pregnant." *CNN*. Cable News Network, February 18, 2014. Web. March 29, 2014.

16   Bitler, Marianne and Lucie Schmidt. "Utilization of Infertility Treatments: The Effects of Insurance Mandates." *Demography* 49.1 (2012): 125–49.

17   Pers. comm. Ms Barbara Collura, President and CEO, RESOLVE, September 22, 2014.

18   Pers. comm. senior official, large health benefit company. February 19, 2014.

19   "GENE.00002 Preimplantation Genetic Diagnosis Testing." Anthem, Inc. 2014.

20   Ibid.

DOI: 10.1057/9781137515445.0007

Bibliography

2012 ART Fertility Clinic Success Rates Report. Rep.: Centers for Disease Control and Prevention, 2014.

Americans with Disabilities Act of 1990. Pub. L. 101–336. July 26, 1990. 104 Stat.

Anticipated Details of the Draft Guidance for Industry, Food and Drug Administration Staff, and Clinical Laboratories. Working paper. Silver Spring, MD: FDA, 2014.

"ASRM/CAP Reproductive Laboratory Accreditation Program." *ASRM Annual Meeting: ASRM/CAP Reproductive Laboratory Accreditation Program Inspector Training Seminar.* N.p., n.d. https://www.asrm.org/ASRM2013_CAP_Course/. Accessed on April 9, 2014.

Asscher, E. C. A. "The Regulation of Preimplantation Genetic Diagnosis (PGD) in the Netherlands and the UK: A Comparative Study of the Regulatory Frameworks and Outcomes for PGD." *Clinical Ethics* 3.4 (2008): 176–179.

Authority Decision on the Use of PGD for Lower Penetrance, Later Onset Inherited Disorders. Rep.: Human Fertilisation and Embryology Authority, 2006.

Baruch, S. "Preimplantation Genetic Diagnosis and Parental Preferences: Beyond Deadly Disease." *Houston Journal of Health Law & Policy* 8 (2009): 245–270.

Baruch, S. "PGD: Genetic Testing of Embryos in the United States." *JRC European Commission.* Johns Hopkins University, February 15, 2009. http://ec.europa.eu/dgs/jrc/downloads/jrc_aaas_2009_03_baruch_pgd.pdf. Accessed on January 26, 2014.

DOI: 10.1057/9781137515445.0008

Baruch, S., D. Kaufman, and K. Hudson. "Genetic Testing of Embryos: Practices and Perspectives of US *In Vitro* Fertilization Clinics." *Fertility and Sterility* 89.5 (2008): 1053–1058.

Baruch, S., G. Javitt, J. Scott, and K. Hudson. *Preimplantation Genetic Diagnosis: A Discussion of Challenges, Concerns, and Preliminary Policy Options Related to the Genetic Testing of Human Embryos.* Washington, DC: Genetics and Public Policy Center, 2004.

Batzer, Frances R. and Vardit Ravitsky, "Preimplantation Genetic Diagnosis: Ethical Considerations," in *The Penn Center Guide to Bioethics.* V. Ravitsky, A. Fiester, and A. L. Caplan, eds. New York: Springer Publishing Co., 2009.

Berkowitz, Jonathan M. and Jack W. Snyder. "Racism and Sexism in Medically Assisted Conception." *Bioethics* 12.1 (1998): 25–44.

Beyond Therapy: Biotechnology and the Pursuit of Happiness: A Report of the President's Council on Bioethics. Washington, DC: President's Council on Bioethics, 2003.

Bitler, Marianne and Lucie Schmidt. "Utilization of Infertility Treatments: The Effects of Insurance Mandates." *Demography* 49.1 (2012): 125–149.

Boss, Emily F., John K. Niparko, Darrell J. Gaskin, and Kimberly L. Levinson. "Socioeconomic Disparities for Hearing-Impaired Children in the United States." *The Laryngoscope* 121.4 (2011): 860–866.

Braude, Peter, Susan Pickering, Frances Flinter, and Caroline Mackie Ogilvie. "Preimplantation Genetic Diagnosis." *Nature Reviews Genetics* 3.12 (2002): 941–955.

"Briefing on HFEA Bill." *Welcome to the RCOG.* Royal College of Obstetricians and Gynaecologists, n.d. Web. October 23, 2013.

Brock, Dan W. "Shaping Future Children: Parental Rights and Societal Interests." *Journal of Political Philosophy* 13.4 (2005): 377–398.

Buchanan, Allen E., Dan W. Brock, Norman Daniels, and Daniel Wikler. *From Chance to Choice: Genetics and Justice.* Cambridge, UK: Cambridge UP, 2000.

Cigna Medical Coverage Policy Preimplantation Genetic Diagnosis. Cigna. October 15, 2013.

Choices and Boundaries: A Summary of Responses to the HFEA Public Discussion. Rep.: Human Fertilisation and Embryology Authority, 2006.

Christensen, Jen. "Record Number of Women Using IVF to Get Pregnant." *CNN.* Cable News Network, February 18, 2014. http://www.cnn.com/2014/02/17/health/record-ivf-use/. March 29, 2014.

DOI: 10.1057/9781137515445.0008

Christman, John. "Autonomy in Moral and Political Philosophy." *Stanford Encyclopedia of Philosophy.* Stanford University, July 28, 2003. http://seop.illc.uva.nl/archives/fall2008/entries/autonomy-moral/. Accessed on February 21, 2014.

"Clinical Decision-Making." *HFEA Guidance on Preimplantation Genetic Testing.* Human Fertilisation and Embryology Authority, 2006. March 22, 2014.

Collins, Francis and Margaret Hamburg. "First FDA Authorization for Next-Generation Sequencer." *New England Journal of Medicine* 369.25 (2013).

Colls, P., L. Silver, G. Olivera, J. Weier, T. Escudero, N. Goodall, G. Tomkin, and S. Munné. "Preimplantation Genetic Diagnosis for Gender Selection in the USA." *Reproductive BioMedicine Online* 19 (2009): 16–22.

Committee on Ethics of the American Congress of Obstetricians and Gynecologists. "Sex Selection." Number 360, February 2007.

Committee on Genetics of the American Congress of Obstetricians and Gynecologists. "Preimplantation Genetic Screening for Aneuploidy." Number 430, March 2009.

Committee on Genetics of the American Congress of Obstetricians and Gynecologists. "Technology Assessment: Genetics and Molecular Diagnostic Testing." Number 11, Febryary 2014.

Committee on Health Care for Underserved Women of the American Congress of Obstetricians and Gynecologists. "Abortion Access and Training: Committee Opinion." Number 424, January 2009.

Committees on Ethics and Genetics of the American Congress of Obstetricians and Gynecologists. "Ethical Issues in Genetic Testing." Number 410, June 2008.

Connecticut Medicaid: Summary of Services. Medical Care Administration Department of Social Services, Connecticut Department of Social Services.

"The Costs of Infertility Treatment." *RESOLVE: The National Infertility Association.* RESOLVE, n.d. http://www.resolve.org/family-building-options/insurance_coverage/the-costs-of-infertility-treatment.html. Accessed on September 19, 2014.

Darnovsky, Marcy. "A Slippery Slope to Human Germline Modification." *Nature* 499.7457 (2013): 127.

Davis, Dena. "Genetic Dilemmas and the Child's Right to an Open Future." *Hastings Center Report* 27.2 (1997): 7–15.

DOI: 10.1057/9781137515445.0008

Edlund, Lena, Hongbin Li, Junjian Yi, and Junsen Zhang. "Sex Ratios and Crime: Evidence from China." *The Review of Economics and Statistics* 95.5 (2013): 1520–1534.

"Egg Retrieval and Embryo Transfer." *Preparing for Egg Retrieval.* Yale Fertility Center, n.d. http://medicine.yale.edu/obgyn/yfc/ourservices/invitro/egg-retrieval.aspx. Accessed on January 26, 2014.

Egnew, Thomas. "The Meaning of Healing: Transcending Suffering." *Annals of Family Medicine* 3.3 (2005): 255–262.

"Essential Health Benefits Standards: Ensuring Quality, Affordable Coverage." Centers for Medicare and Medicaid Services, February 20, 2013. http://www.cms.gov/CCIIO/Resources/Fact-Sheets-and-FAQs/ehb-2-20-2013.html. Accessed on January 26, 2014.

Ethics Committee of the American Society for Reproductive Medicine. "Sex Selection and Preimplantation Genetic Diagnosis." *Fertility and Sterility* 72.4 (1999): 595–598.

Ethics Committee of the American Society for Reproductive Medicine. "Preconception Gender Selection for Nonmedical Reasons." *Fertility and Sterility* 75.5 (2001): 861–864.

Ethics Committee of the American Society for Reproductive Medicine. "Use of Preimplantation Genetic Diagnosis for Serious Adult Onset Conditions: A Committee Opinion." *Fertility and Sterility* 100 (2013): 54–57.

Fallon, Jr. Richard H. "Two Senses of Autonomy." *Stanford Law Review* 46.4 (1994): 875–905.

Feinberg, Joel. "The Child's Right to an Open Future." *Whose Child? Children's Rights, Parental Authority, and State Power.* Totowa, New Jersey: Littlefield, Adams & Co, 1980. Pages 124–153.

"The Fertility Clinic Success Rate and Certification Act." *Policy Documents.* Centers for Disease Control and Prevention, October 31, 2013. http://www.cdc.gov/art/Policy.htm. Accessed on April 08, 2014.

Fossett, James W., Alicia R. Ouellette, Sean Philpott, David Magnus, and Glenn McGee. "Federalism and Bioethics: States and Moral Pluralism." *Hastings Center Report* 37.6 (2007): 24–35.

Francis, Leslie Pickering and Anita Silvers. "A Wrongful Case for Parental Tort Liability." *The American Journal of Bioethics* 12.4 (2012): 15–17.

Fryhofer, Sandra. *Is Obesity a Disease.* Rep. Vol. 3-A-13. American Medical Association, 2013. Report of the Council on Science and Public Health.

DOI: 10.1057/9781137515445.0008

Gallagher, J. "Preimplantation Genetic Diagnosis for IVF 'Is Safe'"
BBC News. BBC, March 7, 2012. http://www.bbc.co.uk/news/health-
18676894. Accessed on January 26, 2014.

Galton, Francis. "Eugenics: Its Definition, Scope, and Aims." *American
Journal of Sociology* 10.1 (1904): 1–25.

Gaylin, Willard and Bruce Jennings. *The Perversion of Autonomy:
Coercion and Constraints in a Liberal Society,* 2nd ed., Washington, DC:
Georgetown University Press, 2004.

"GENE.00002 Preimplantation Genetic Diagnosis Testing." Anthem,
Inc., October 8, 2013. http://www.anthem.com/medicalpolicies/
policies/mp_pw_a049872.htm. Accessed on March 29, 2014.

Genetic Information Nondiscrimination Act of 2008. H.R. 493, 110
Cong., Congressional Record (2008) (enacted).

Genetics and Human Behaviour: The Ethical Context. Rep. London:
Nuffield Council on Bioethics, 2002.

Gianaroli, Luca, Anna Maria Crivello, Ilaria Stanghellini, Anna Pia
Ferraretti, Carla Tabanelli, and Maria Cristina Magli. "Reiterative
Changes in the Italian Regulation on IVF: The Effect on PGD
Patients' Reproductive Decisions." *Reproductive BioMedicine Online*
28.1 (2013): 125–132.

Grody, Wayne, Barry H. Thompson, Anthony R. Gregg, Lora H. Bean,
Kristin G. Monaghan, Adele Schneider, and Roger V. Lebo. "ACMG
Position Statement on Prenatal/Preconception Expanded Carrier
Screening." American College of Medical Genetics and Genomics.
Genetics in Medicine 15.5 (2013): 482–483.

Gutierrez, Alberto. "Warning Letter to 23andMe, Inc." *Inspections,
Compliance, Enforcement, and Criminal Investigations.* Food and Drug
Administration, November 22, 2013. http://www.fda.gov/ICECI/
EnforcementActions/WarningLetters/2013/ucm376296.htm. Accessed
on March 14, 2014.

Harris, John. *Enhancing Evolution: The Ethical Case for Making Better
People.* Princeton, NJ: Princeton UP, 2007.

HFEA Standing Orders. Rep.: Human Fertilisation and Embryology
Authority, 2013.

Hippocrates. "The Hippocratic Oath." *Greek Medicine.* Trans. Michael
North. U.S. National Library of Medicine, July 2, 2012. https://www.nlm.
nih.gov/hmd/greek/greek_oath.html. Accessed on February 13, 2014.

"How does PGD Work?" *PGD—Preimplantation Genetic Diagnosis
(PGD)—Genetic Testing.* Human Fertilisation and Embryology

DOI: 10.1057/9781137515445.0008

Authority, n.d. http://www.hfea.gov.uk/preimplantation-genetic-diagnosis.html . Accessed on November 28, 2013.

Huang, Jack, Togas Tulandi, Hananel Holzer, Seang Lin Tan, and Ri-Cheng Chian. "Combining Ovarian Tissue Cryobanking with Retrieval of immature Oocytes Followed by *In Vitro* Maturation and Vitrification: An Additional Strategy of Fertility Preservation." *Fertility and Sterility* 89.3 (2008): 567–572.

Hudson, K. "Preimplantation Genetic Diagnosis: Public Policy and Public Attitudes." *Fertility and Sterility* 85.6 (2006): 1638–1645.

Hughes, James. *Citizen Cyborg: Why Democratic Societies Must Respond to the Redesigned Human of the Future.* Cambridge, MA: Westview, 2004.

Human Fertilisation and Embryology Act (as amended). Schedule 2. London, United Kingdom, 1990.

Human Fertilisation and Embryology Bill. Bill 6, House of Lords. United Kingdom, 2007–2008.

"Illumina Launches the NextSeq(TM) 500 Sequencing System." *Wall Street Journal* [New York City] January 14, 2014.

"Implantation and Early Development—Study Group Statement." *Welcome to the RCOG.* Royal College of Obstetricians and Gynaecologists, n.d.

"Infertility." *Clinical Policy Bulletin.* Aetna, February 7, 2014. http://www.aetna.com/cpb/medical/data/300_399/0327.html. Accessed on November 21, 2014.

Infertility Coverage Determination Guideline. United Healthcare. May 1, 2013.

"Invasive Prenatal Diagnosis of Genetic Diseases." *Clinical Policy Bulletin.* Aetna, April 29, 2014. http://www.aetna.com/cpb/medical/data/300_399/0358.html. Accessed on September 19, 2014.

Jennings, Bruce. "Technology and the Genetic Imaginary: Prenatal Testing and the Construction of Disability," in *Prenatal Testing and Disability Rights.* Erik Parens and Adrienne Asch, eds. Washington, DC: Georgetown UP, 2000. Pages 124–144.

Kalfoglou, Andrea, Kathy Hudson, and Joan Scott. "PGD Patients' and Providers' Attitudes to the Use and Regulation of Preimplantation Genetic Diagnosis." *Reproductive BioMedicine Online* 11.4 (2005): 486–496.

Kamm, F. M. *Bioethical Prescriptions to Create, End, Choose, and Improve Lives.* Oxford: Oxford University Press, 2013.

Kant, Immanuel. *The Moral Law, or, Kant's Groundwork of the Metaphysic of Morals: A New Translation with Analysis and Notes.* Trans. H. J. Paton. New York: Barnes & Noble, 1956.

DOI: 10.1057/9781137515445.0008

LaFraniere, Sharon. "Chinese Bias for Baby Boys Creates a Gap of 32 Million." *New York Times,* April 10, 2009.

Lang, Joshua. "What Happens to Women Who Are Denied Abortions?" *The New York Times,* June 12, 2013. http://www. nytimes.com/2013/06/16/magazine/study-women-denied-abortions.html?pagewanted=all&_r=0. Accessed on February 22, 2014.

Latham, Melanie. "Regulating the New Reproductive Technologies: A Cross-Channel Comparison." *Medical Law International* 3 (1998): 89–115.

Leigh, Suzanne. "Reproductive 'Tourism' " *USA Today—Health and Behavior.* USATODAY.com, May 2, 2005. http://usatoday30.usatoday. com/news/health/2005-05-02-reproductive-tourism_x.htm. Accessed on September 19, 2014.

Leslie-Miller, Jana. "From Buck to Bell: Responsible Reproduction in the Twentieth Century." *Maryland Journal of Contemporary Legal Issues* 123.8 (1997): 123–150.

Levi, N. "Deafness, Culture and Choice." *Journal of Medical Ethics* 28.5 (2002): 284–285.

Loi relative à la bioéthique. Loi no. 2011-814. French Parliament, 2011.

Lombardo, Paul A. *Three Generations, No Imbeciles: Eugenics, the Supreme Court, and Buck v. Bell.* Baltimore: Johns Hopkins University Press, 2008.

Malek, Janet and Judith Daar. "The Case for a Parental Duty to Use Preimplantation Genetic Diagnosis for Medical Benefit." *The American Journal of Bioethics* 12.4 (2012): 3–11.

Murray, Thomas H. *The Worth of a Child.* Berkeley: University of California Press, 1996.

Murray, Thomas H., "Stirring the Simmering 'Designer Baby' Pot," *Science* 343 (March 14, 2014): 1208–1210.

New PGD Conditions Licensed by the HFEA between 1 April 2012 and 31 March 2013. Rep. N.p.: Human Fertilisation and Embryology Authority, 2013.

NHS Commissioning Board Clinical Reference Group for Genetics. Clinical Commissioning Policy: Pre-Implantation Genetic Diagnosis (PGD). Rep. N.p.: NHS Commissioning Board, 2013.

"The NHS in England." About the National Health Service (NHS) in England. NHS, n.d. http://www.nhs.uk/NHSEngland/thenhs/about/ Pages/overview.aspx. Accessed on September 19, 2014.

"Obesity Is Now a Disease, American Medical Association Decides."
   Medical News Today. MediLexicon International, August 17, 2013.
   http://www.medicalnewstoday.com/articles/262226.php. Accessed on
   February 26, 2014.

"PGD Conditions Licensed by the HFEA." *Your Treatment and Storage
   Options.* Human Fertilisation and Embryology Authority, n.d. http://
   guide.hfea.gov.uk/pgd/. Accessed on March 22, 2014.

Post, Stephen G. and Peter J. Whitehouse, eds. *Genetic Testing for
   Alzheimer Disease: Ethical and Clinical Issues.* Baltimore: The Johns
   Hopkins University Press, 1998.

Preimplantation Genetic Diagnosis in Europe. Rep. Luxembourg: European
   Commission Joint Research Center, 2007. JRC Scientific and
   Technical Reports.

"Preimplantation Genetic Diagnosis, Testing, and Screening
   Information and FAQ's." *PGD.* IVF1.com, November 3, 2013. http://
   www.ivf1.com/pgd/. Accessed on March 30, 2014.

"Preimplantation Genetic Testing: A Practice Committee Opinion."
   Fertility and Sterility 90.5 (2008): S136–143.

Preimplantation Tissue Typing: Policy Review. Rep.: Human Fertilisation
   and Embryology Authority, 2004.

Reid, T. R. *The Healing of America: A Global Quest for Better, Cheaper, and
   Fairer Health Care.* New York: Penguin, 2009.

*Reproduction and Responsibility: The Regulation of New Biotechnologies:
   A Report of the President's Council on Bioethics.* Washington, DC:
   President's Council on Bioethics, 2004.

"Reproductive Genetic Testing in the United States—A Regulatory
   Patchwork." *Genetics & Public Policy Center International Law Search.*
   Genetics & Public Policy Center, January 2004. http://www.
   dnapolicy.org/policy.international.php?action=detail&laws_
   id=63. Accessed on October 23, 2013.

"Risks of *In Vitro* Fertilization (IVF)." *ASRM Patient Fact Sheet.* American
   Society for Reproductive Medicine, n.d. http://www.asrm.org/
   Risks_of_In_Vitro_Fertilization_factsheet/. Accessed on April 1, 2014.

Robertson, John. "Assisting Reproduction, Choosing Genes and the
   Scope of Reproductive Autonomy." *The George Washington Law Review*
   76.6 (2008): 1490–1513.

Rodwin, Marc A. *Conflicts of Interest and the Future of Medicine: The
   United States, France, and Japan.* Oxford, England: Oxford University
   Press, 2011.

DOI: 10.1057/9781137515445.0008

Saad, Lydia. "Americans' Abortion Views Steady Amid Gosnell Trial." Gallup.com, May 10, 2013. http://www.gallup.com/poll/162374/ americans-abortion-views-steady-amid-gosnell-trial.aspx. Accessed on March 17, 2014.

Sandel, Michael J. *The Case against Perfection: Ethics in the Age of Genetic Engineering*. Cambridge, MA: Belknap of Harvard UP, 2007.

Sandel, Michael J. "The Case against Perfection." *Atlantic Monthly* 293.3 (2004): 51–62.

Savulescu, Julian. "Procreative Beneficence: Why We Should Select the Best Children." *Bioethics* 15.5–6 (2001): 413–426.

Saxton, Marsha. "Why Members of the Disability Community Oppose Prenatal Diagnosis and Selective Abortion," in *Prenatal Testing and Disability Rights*. Erik Parens and Adrienne Asch, eds. Washington, DC: Georgetown UP, 2000. Pages 147–164.

Scott, Rosamund. *Choosing between Possible Lives*. Oxford: Hart, 2007.

Simpson, Joe, Robert Rebar, and Sandra Carson. "Professional Self-Regulation for Preimplantation Genetic Diagnosis: Experience of the American Society for Reproductive Medicine and Other Professional Societies." *Fertility and Sterility* 85 (2006): 1653–1660.

Spar, Debora L. *The Baby Business: How Money, Science, and Politics Drive the Commerce of Conception*. Boston: Harvard Business School, 2006.

Stankovic, Bratislav. " 'It's a Designer Baby!'—Opinions on Regulation of Preimplantation Genetic Diagnosis." *UCLA Journal of Law and Technology* 3 (2005): n. pag.

"State Laws Related to Insurance Coverage for Infertility Treatment." *Insurance Coverage for Infertility Laws*. National Conference of State Legislatures, June 2014. http://www.ncsl.org/issues-research/health/ insurance-coverage-for-infertility-laws.aspx. Accessed on September 19, 2014.

Thornhill, A. R. "ESHRE PGD Consortium 'Best Practice Guidelines for Clinical Preimplantation Genetic Diagnosis (PGD) and Preimplantation Genetic Screening (PGS)' " *Human Reproduction* 20.1 (2004): 35–48.

Ubel, Peter. "Are Infertility Doctors Turning into Predatory Bankers?" *Forbes*. Forbes Magazine, December 11, 2012. http://www.forbes. com/sites/peterubel/2012/12/11/are-infertility-doctors-turning-into-predatory-bankers/. Accessed on September 22, 2014.

DOI: 10.1057/9781137515445.0008

"Vaccines, Blood & Biologics: Compliance Program Guidance Manual." *Tissue & Tissue Products*. Food and Drug Administration, n.d. Web. March 14, 2014.

Von Hagel, Alison. "Banking on Infertility: Medical Ethics and the Marketing of Fertility Loans." *Hastings Center Report* 43.6 (2013): 15–17.

Wilkinson, Stephen. *Choosing Tomorrow's Children: The Ethics of Selective Reproduction*. Oxford, England: Clarendon, 2010.

Wilson, Robert. "Environmental Regulation of the Human Gene Pool as a Genetic Commons." *N.Y.U. Environmental Law Journal* 5 (1996): 833–857.

Wolf, Susan, Jeffrey Kahn, and John Wagner. "Using Preimplantation Genetic Diagnosis to Create a Stem Cell Donor: Issues, Guidelines & Limits." *Journal of Law, Medicine and Ethics* 31 (2003): 327–339.

Yost, Judith. *CLIA and Genetic Testing Oversight*. Rep.: Center for Medicare and Medicaid Services, 2008.

Interviews (in chronological order):

1 Dr Mark Hughes, Founder and Director of Genesis Genetics. January 15, 2014. Phone.

2 Dr Paula Amato, Chair, Ethics Committee of the American Society for Reproductive Medicine. January 16, 2014. Phone.

3 Dr Santiago Munné, Founder and Director of Reprogenetics. January 21, 2014. E-mail.

4 Ms Barbara Collura, President and CEO, RESOLVE. February 4, 2014. Phone.

5 Prof. Anita Silvers, Chair of Philosophy, San Francisco State University. February 8, 2014. Phone.

6 Prof. Laura Mauldin, Women's, Gender and Sexuality Studies, University of Connecticut. February 10, 2014. E-mail.

7 Prof. Leslie Francis, Law and Philosophy, University of Utah. February 14, 2014. Phone.

8 Ms Alison Lashwood, Clinical Lead in PGD, Centre for Preimplantation Genetic Diagnosis, Guy's and St Thomas' Hospital, London, UK. March 26, 2014. Phone.

DOI: 10.1057/9781137515445.0008

Index

abortion, 2, 3, 9, 26, 60, 61, 69, 73
adult-onset diseases, 8–9, 50–2
Aetna, 90–1
Affordable Care Act, 13
Agence de la Biomédecine, 12
Alzheimer's disease, 8, 16n25, 51
Amato, P., 74
American College of Medical Genetics (ACMG), 11, 69, 73, 76–7
American Congress of Obstetricians and Gynecologists (ACOG), 11, 69, 73, 75–6
American Medical Association (AMA), 41, 42
American Society for Reproductive Medicine (ASRM), 6, 11, 16n24, 43, 69, 71, 73–5, 77–9, 93
American with Disabilities Act, 45
aneuploidy screening, see preimplantation chromosomal screening (PGS)
Anthem PGD policy, 94–5
assisted reproductive technology (ART), 8, 60, 77, 90, 93
  annual report, 70
  laws related to, 72
  regulation of, 11–13, 29

Baruch, S., 7, 8, 20, 28
BRCA breast cancer genes, 41, 74
breast cancer, 8, 9, 41, 44
Brock, D., 27
Buck v. Bell, 60–1, 66

Caplan, A., 11
Centers for Disease Control and Prevention (CDC), 6, 69, 70–1
Centers for Medicare and Medicaid Services (CMS), 69, 71
Clinical Laboratory Improvement Amendments (CLIA), 71
coercion, 65–7, 84n28
Collins, F., 5
Collura, B., 93–4
cryopreservation, 5–6, 15n11
cystic fibrosis, 2, 3, 7, 8, 43, 49, 50, 76

Daar, J., 33–4, 40
Davis, D., 30, 45, 48, 62
deafness, 10, 12
  negative impact of, on children, 45–6
  perceptions of, 45–6
  selection against, 34, 41, 44–7, 67
  selection for, 4, 7, 48–50, 62–3, 75

DOI: 10.1057/9781137515445.0009

Department of Veterans Affairs
system, 12–13
"designer babies", 29–30, 32, 34, 40, 73,
96–7
disability, 7–8, 10, 30, 34, 40–2, 45–51,
55, 62–3, 67–9, 78, 80 95
disease
definitions of, 40–3
harm and, 42–3
serious/severe, 34, 40, 42–4
and use of PGD, 40–4
donor sibling, 53–4
dwarfism, 4, 10, 12, 67, 84n27

ethical controversies, 7–10
eugenics
authoritarian, 65–6
coercive, 66, 67, 84n24
definitions of, 65–6
and implications for PGD, 65–8
'laissez-faire', 65, 84n24
negative, 66–7
positive, 66–7
expressivist argument, 46–7, 51, 52, 64,
67

Feinberg, J., 30, 62
Fertility Clinic Success Rate and
Certification Act (FCSRA), 70
Food and Drug Administration (FDA),
5, 69–70
France, 11–13

genetic determinism, 27, 51
Genetic Information
Nondiscrimination Act
(GINA), 92
Genetics and Public Policy Center
(GPPC), 7, 10
genetic selection, 26–8, 30, 31, 34,
37n31, 43, 67
genetic sequencing technology, 5
see also Illumina, Inc. gene
sequencer
genetic technology, 3, 7, 27, 40
Griswold v. Connecticut, 61

Hamburg, M., 5
harm
and disease, 42–3
non-person-affecting,
49–50
person-affecting, 49
Harris, J., 20
HiSeq X sequencer, 5
Hudson, K., 7
Hughes, J., 20
human dignity, 8, 52–3
Human Fertilisation and Embryology
Authority (HFEA), 11, 13, 71–2,
79–81, 94, 95
Human Leukocyte Antigen (HLA)
typing/matching, 4, 7, 8, 53, 74
humility, 20–4, 29, 32, 36n13, 37n30, 43,
48, 49, 64
Huntington's disease, 8–9, 49, 50, 51
hyperstimulation, of ovaries, 6, 23

Illumina, Inc. gene sequencer, 5, 70
infertility, 2, 5, 11, 13–14, 77–8, 82, 90–1,
93–4
in vitro fertilization (IVF), 2–5, 29,
42–3, 70
costs, 90
cycle/cycles, 4, 6, 7, 14, 40, 71,
90, 93
effect of, 16n24
health insurance coverage for, 13, 14,
64, 90–5

Joint Commission on Accreditation
of Healthcare Organizations
(JCAHO), 71

Kamm, F., 21, 25, 35n13
Kaufman, D., 7

Malek, J., 33–4, 40
mastery, 20–2
Mauldin, L., 45, 46
Medicaid, 12, 13, 72
Medicare, 12, 13, 72
MiSeqDx system, 5

National Health Insurance (NHI), 13
National Health Service (NHS), 11, 13, 72
NextSeq 500 System, 5
nonidentity problem, 10, 32, 38n39, 49–50, 62

obesity, 41, 42

parenthood/parenting/parents
  and commodification of children, 28–9
  control of vs. autonomy of the future child, 29–31, 37n32
  humility as the basis of, 20–3
  and the norm of unconditional love, 24–6
  over-the-top attitudes of, 26–7
  and "right to an open future" argument, 30–1, 48–9, 62
  and selfishness, 28
Parkinson's disease, 51
preimplantation chromosomal screening (PGS), 5, 7, 76
preimplantation genetic diagnosis (PGD)
  costs, 90
  and creation of savior siblings, 52–4
  ethical critique of, 20–4
  future areas of research on, 97–8
  government regulation vs. self-regulation of, 77–9
  health care funding and coverage of, 12–14, 72, 78, 90–5
  and HLA matching controversy, 8
  and impact on parent–child relationship, 24–5
  implications of eugenics for, 65–8
  Kamm's perspectives on, 21–2, 35n13
  limitations of, 6, 31, 34
  medical purposes of, 2–4, 8–9, 11
  medical–nonmedical distinctions of, 23–4, 67
  moral gray zones and, 34, 44, 79–81
  and moral obligation to use, 32–4

nonmedical uses of, 4–5, 9–10, 33, 40, 54, 63, 67, 81–2
  options for government regulation of, 68–73
  public and specialist opinions on regulation of, 81–3, 88n79
  practice in the United States, overview, 6–7
  procedure, 4–6
  and regulatory flexibility, 79–81
  relevance of 'disease' concept to the use of, 40–4
  Sandel's opinions on, *see* Sandel, M.
  Savulescu's views on, 31–4
  and selection, *see* selection
  and sex selection, *see* sex selection
  and state legislatures, 72–3
President's Council on Bioethics, 43–4
"Procreative Beneficence" principle, 32–3

reproductive autonomy, 55
  cases illustrative of, 60–2
  and eugenics, 68
  and the gene pool concept, 64–5
  limitations of, 60–5, 66, 68
  and state interests in regulation, 62–5
  state legislatures and, 72–3
reproductive freedom, 45, 60, 65, 68, 69
reproductive rights, 48, 55, 60–1, 97
RESOLVE, 93–4
right to an open future, 30–1, 48–9, 62
Robertson, J., 61–2
Roe v. Wade, 61

Sandel, M.
  criticisms on the views of, 21, 25–7, 35n13
  on healing vs. enhancing, 22–4, 43
  on humility as the basis for parenthood, 20–3
  on over-the-top parenting attitudes, 26–7

Sandel, M. – *continued*
  on parent–child relationship, 24–5
  on selfishness in parents, 28
savior sibling, 4, 8, 52–4
Savulescu, J., 20
  on disease, 40
  on disability, 46, 57n24
  on "Procreative Beneficence"
    concept, 32–4
Scott, R., 45
selection
  against adult-onset diseases, 8–9,
    50–2
  against autosomal recessive
    polycystic kidney disease
    (ARPKD), 34
  against deafness, 44–7
  for deafness, 48–50
  for a disability, 10
  positive, 27, 67
  negative, 27, 41–3, 45, 47, 64, 67
  sex, *see* sex selection
  for/against traits, 4–5, 7–8, 10
self-regulation of, 11–12, 73–7
sex selection

ACOG Ethics Committee Opinion
    on, 75–6
  elective, 4–5, 7, 9–10, 11, 54–6, 63
  for family balancing, 54–5
  and gender bias, 9–10, 32, 54–5
  nonmedical, 7–10, 12, 32, 50, 55, 64
  and parental preference, 54–5
sex stereotyping, 54
sex supremacy, 54
Skinner v. Oklahoma, 60–1
Society for Assisted Reproductive
    Technology (SART), 6–7

Tay-Sachs disease, 2, 7, 8, 43,
    52, 67

United Healthcare, 90
United Kingdom, 11, 13
US Congress, 69, 71
utilitarian, 32–4, 38n40, 57n24

Virginia Sterilization Act (1924), 66

whole-genome sequencing, 5, 6
Wilkinson, S., 54, 65

DOI: 10.1057/9781137515445.0009